Joseph Meites

COMPARATIVE ENDOCRINOLOGY OF PROLACTIN

ADVANCES IN EXPERIMENTAL MEDICINE AND BIOLOGY

Editorial Board:

Nathan Back	State University of New York at Buffalo
N. R. Di Luzio	Tulane University School of Medicine
Bernard Halpern	Collège de France and Institute of Immuno-Biology
Ephraim Katchalski	The Weizmann Institute of Science
David Kritchevsky	Wistar Institute
Abel Lajtha	New York State Research Institute for Neurochemistry and Drug Addiction
Rodolfo Paoletti	University of Milan

Recent Volumes in this Series

Volume 79
ELASTIN AND ELASTIC TISSUE
Edited by Lawrence B. Sandberg, William R. Gray, and Carl Franzblau • 1977

Volume 80
COMPARATIVE ENDOCRINOLOGY OF PROLACTIN
Edited by Horst-Dieter Dellmann, J. Alan Johnson, and David M. Klachko • 1977

Volume 81
PHOSPHATE METABOLISM
Edited by Shaul G. Massry and Eberhard Ritz • 1977

Volume 82
ATHEROSCLEROSIS: Metabolic, Morphologic, and Clinical Aspects
Edited by George W. Manning and M. Daria Haust • 1977

Volume 83
FUNCTION AND BIOSYNTHESIS OF LIPIDS
Edited by Nicolás G. Bazán, Rodolfo R. Brenner, and Norma M. Giusto • 1977

Volume 84
MEMBRANE TOXICITY
Edited by Morton W. Miller and Adil E. Shamoo • 1977

Volume 85A
ALCOHOL INTOXICATION AND WITHDRAWAL – IIIa: Biological Effects of Alcohol
Edited by Milton M. Gross • 1977

Volume 85B
ALCOHOL INTOXICATION AND WITHDRAWAL – IIIb: Studies in Alcohol Dependence
Edited by Milton M. Gross • 1977

Volume 86A
PROTEIN CROSSLINKING: Biochemical and Molecular Aspects
Edited by Mendel Friedman • 1977

Volume 86B
PROTEIN CROSSLINKING: Nutritional and Medical Consequences
Edited by Mendel Friedman • 1977

COMPARATIVE ENDOCRINOLOGY OF PROLACTIN

Edited by
Horst-Dieter Dellmann
Iowa State University
Ames, Iowa

J. Alan Johnson
and
David M. Klachko
University of Missouri
Columbia, Missouri

PLENUM PRESS • NEW YORK AND LONDON

Library of Congress Cataloging in Publication Data

Midwest Conference on Endocrinology and Metabolism, 10th, University of Missouri—Columbia, 1974.
Comparative endocrinology of prolactin.

(Advances in experimental medicine and biology; v. 80)
Proceedings of a conference sponsored by the University of Missouri—Columbia, and others.

Includes index.

1. Lactogenic hormones—Congresses. I. Dellmann, Horst-Dieter. II. Johnson, Joseph Alan, 1933-   III. Klachko, David M. IV. University of Missouri—Columbia. V. Title. VI. Series. [DNLM: 1. Prolactin—Metabolism—Congresses. 2. Physiology, Comparative—Congresses. AD559 v. 80 1974/WK515 M629c 1974] 1974/WK515 M629c 1974]
QP572.L3M5 1974   599'.01'927   77-1871
ISBN 0-306-39080-9

Proceedings of the Tenth Midwest Conference on Endocrinology and Metabolism held at the University of Missouri, Columbia, Missouri, October 3—4, 1974 and sponsored by

    University of Missouri - Columbia
        College of Agriculture
        Dalton Research Center
        Division of Biological Sciences
        Extension Division
        Graduate School
        School of Medicine
        Sinclair Comparative Medicine Research Farm
    American Chemical Society - UMC Section
    Ayerst Laboratories
    Ciba-Geigy Corporation
    Merck, Sharp, and Dohme
    Organon Incorporated
    Searle Laboratories, G.D. Searle & Co.
    The Squibb Institute of Medical Research

© 1977 Plenum Press, New York
A Division of Plenum Publishing Corporation
227 West 17th Street, New York, N.Y. 10011

All rights reserved

No part of this book may be reproduced, stored in a retrieval system, or transmitted, in any form or by any means, electronic, mechanical, photocopying, microfilming, recording, or otherwise, without written permission from the Publisher

Printed in the United States of America

Conference Chairman

DAVID M. KLACHKO, M.D., Associate Professor of Medicine, University of Missouri - Columbia

Planning Committee

CONSTANTINE S. ANAST, M.D., Professor of Pediatrics, University of Missouri - Columbia

RALPH R. ANDERSON, Ph.D., Associate Professor of Dairy Husbandry, University of Missouri - Columbia

HORST-DIETER DELLMANN, Dr. vet. med., Ph.D., Professor of Veterinary Anatomy, University of Missouri - Columbia

LEONARD R. FORTE, Ph.D., Assistant Professor of Pharmacology, University of Missouri - Columbia

JOHN M. FRANZ, Ph.D., Associate Professor of Biochemistry, University of Missouri - Columbia

JAMES A. GREEN, Ph.D., Professor of Anatomy, University of Missouri - Columbia

LAURENCE W. HEDLUND, Ph.D., Assistant Professor of Dairy Husbandry, University of Missouri - Columbia

RONALD C. JAMES, M.D., Assistant Professor of Medicine, University of Missouri - Columbia

J. ALAN JOHNSON, Ph.D., Assistant Professor of Physiology, University of Missouri - Columbia

BARBARA MAIER, Conference Coordinator, Conferences and Short Courses, University Extension Division, University of Missouri - Columbia

WARREN L. ZAHLER, Ph.D., Assistant Professor of Agricultural Chemistry, University of Missouri - Columbia

Speakers

MARILYN G. FARQUHAR, Ph.D., Professor of Cell Biology and Pathology, Yale University School of Medicine, New Haven, Connecticut

ANDREW G. FRANTZ, M.D., Professor of Medicine, College of Physicians and Surgeons of Columbia University, New York, New York

LAURENCE S. JACOBS, M.D., Assistant Professor of Medicine, Washington University School of Medicine, St. Louis, Missouri

URBAN J. LEWIS, Ph.D., Endocrine Division, Scripps Clinic and Research Foundation, La Jolla, California

ALBERT H. MEIER, Ph.D., Professor of Zoology and Physiology, Louisiana State University, Baton Rouge, Louisiana

JOSEPH MEITES, Ph.D., Professor of Physiology, Michigan State University, East Lansing, Michigan

CHARLES W. TURNER, Ph.D., Professor Emeritus of Dairy Husbandry, University of Missouri - Columbia

Additional Speakers

GARY C. BOND, Ph.D., Assistant Professor of Physiology and Biophysics, University of Arkansas, Little Rock, Arkansas

JAMES N. PASLEY, Ph.D., Associate Professor of Physiology and Biophysics, University of Arkansas, Little Rock, Arkansas

THOMAS I. KOIKE, Ph.D., Associate Professor of Physiology and Biophysics, University of Arkansas, Little Rock, Arkansas

Moderators

RALPH R. ANDERSON, Ph.D., Associate Professor of Dairy Husbandry, University of Missouri - Columbia

WARREN R. FLEMING, Ph.D., Professor of Biological Sciences, University of Missouri - Columbia

JAMES A. GREEN, Ph.D., Professor of Anatomy, University of Missouri - Columbia

JOHN L. WINNACKER, M.D., Assistant Professor of Medicine, University of Missouri - Columbia

Discussants

BARNAWELL, E.B., School of Life Sciences, University of Nebraska - Lincoln, Nebraska

DELLMANN, H.-D., Department of Veterinary Anatomy and Physiology, University of Missouri - Columbia

DERBY, A., Department of Biology, University of Missouri - St. Louis

FLEMING, W.R., Division of Biological Sciences, University of Missouri - Columbia

GILLESPIE, R.L., 5125 Rondel Place, Columbia, Maryland

KLEIN, T.A., L.A. County Hospital, University of Southern California, Los Angeles, California

MILLS, J.B., Department of Biochemistry, Emory University, Atlanta, Georgia

PARSONS, J.A., Department of Anatomy, University of Minnesota, Minneapolis, Minnesota

SAGE, M., Department of Biology, University of Missouri - St. Louis

WINNACKER, J.L., Department of Medicine, University of Missouri - Columbia

PREFACE

The selection of prolactin as the subject of the Midwest Conference on Endocrinology was not only dictated by the recent advances in prolactin research but also by the long tradition in that particular area of Endocrinology in the laboratory of C.W. Turner at the University of Missouri. Therefore, it seems only appropriate that these proceedings of the Tenth Midwest Conference on Endocrinology are dedicated to the memory of this scientist, deceased in August 1975 before completion of this volume, whose pioneer investigations have contributed substantially to the advancement of our knowledge in many areas of Endocrinology and who played a major role in the early phases of prolactin research.

This volume contains a review of the early studies in Turner's laboratory and the latest results obtained by some of the leading research workers in this area and should be a fitting memory to C.W. Turner.

Some of the manuscripts printed here were prepared after the conference was held and include material of more recent origin. Much of the delay in publication was due to the length of time devoted to preparation of these manuscripts. To the other authors and participants, and to Plenum Press, we express our appreciation for their patience and cooperation. We also with to thank Mrs. Katherine Browning, Mrs. Susan Haines, and Mrs. Linda Bennett for their sterling efforts in helping prepare the proceedings for publication. Of course, without the efforts of the Planning Committee and the contributions of the sponsors, there would have been no conference.

H.-Dieter Dellmann
J. Alan Johnson
David M. Klachko

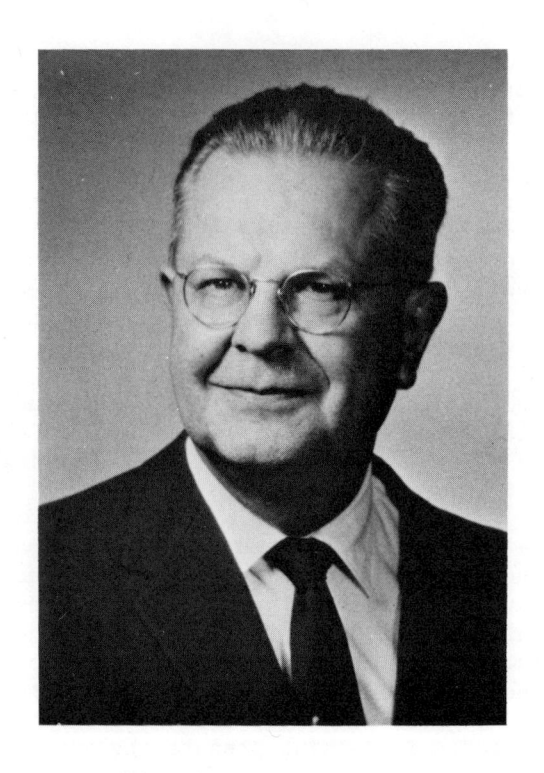

Dr. Charles W. Turner

MEMORIAL TO DR. CHARLES W. TURNER

This volume of the Proceedings of the 10th Midwest Conference on Endocrinology and Metabolism is dedicated to Dr. Charles W. Turner, who passed away on August 25, 1975. Dr. Turner's interest in prolactin as a principal hormonal control of breast development and lactation spanned a period of five decades from 1925 to 1975.

In the early years of his career, Dr. Turner's interests were centered upon the composition of milk and factors, both genetic and environmental, which influenced composition and quantity of milk. During the period of study and research at the University of Wisconsin toward the Ph.D. degree, he became interested in the embryonic and fetal development of the mammary gland (breast) in cattle. The results of this study and the influences by endocrinological zoologists at Wisconsin, including Hisaw and Fevold, generated enthusiasm for linking the endocrines with genetics in understanding physiological mechanisms related to high milk production. While he was conducting studies on the relation of estrogens to mammary development in the late twenties, Dr. Turner became aware of the newly published work of Stricker and Grueter demonstrating the presence of an anterior pituitary hormone responsible for initiation and maintenance of lactation.

While he was still very much in the midst of research describing the role of estrogens in mammary growth, Dr. Turner assigned his new graduate student, W.U. Gardner, to the task of identifying the anterior pituitary factor responsible for lactation. The result of Dr. Gardner's work was the bioassay for prolactin we know as the pseudopregnant rabbit assay. On day 16 of pseudopregnancy in the rabbit, the mammary gland is developed to the extent that the adenohypophysial hormone prolactin will initiate milk synthesis in the epithelial cells of previously formed alveolar structures.

Since Dr. Gardner's assay was qualitative, and not quantitative, the research group under Dr. Turner's direction wanted to find a quantitative assay for the anterior pituitary hormone responsible for lactation. Incidentally, Drs. Turner and Gardner named this hormone galactin. When the name was not universally accepted, Dr. Turner accepted the name lactogenic hormone or lactogen, but not prolactin, a word originated by Riddle and Bates. These investigators also developed the only good quantitative bioassay available to researchers on prolactin, the pigeon crop assay. Several of Dr. Turner's students and colleagues improved upon the pigeon crop assay over the years to make it more sensitive than it had been previously. These men included Dr. W.H. McShan, Dr. R.P. Reece, and Dr. C.E. Grosvenor.

An early observation of Dr. Turner was the ability of estrogens to stimulate ductal growth in the mammary gland, while progesterone was more effective in stimulating lobule-alveolar growth. This was followed by evidence in conjunction with Dr. Gomez on hypophysectomized animals indicating that steroid hormones were not in themselves mammogenic, but required the synergistic action of the adenohypophysial hormone of Stricker and Grueter. From these observations, Dr. Turner originated the mammogen hypothesis. This stated that a hormone of adenohypophysial origin synergized with estrogens during estrous cycles and in early pregnancy to stimulate duct growth of the mammary apparatus. This hormone was named mammogen I by Dr. Turner. The second hormone of the anterior lobe of the pituitary synergized with progesterone to stimulate lobule-alveolar growth of the gland. This was called mammogen II. Work on this hypothesis led to some interesting physiological findings concerning the mammary gland, but biochemical evidence supports the concept of prolactin being a homologous protein species which is responsible for both mammogenic and lactogenic actions.

During the late forties, several investigators demonstrated the constancy of DNA per cell nucleus in most somatic cells of the body. This concept was immediately adapted by Dr. Turner and his postdoctoral associate, Dr. W.M. Kirkham, and a long sought-after solution to the problem of assessing mammary development quantitatively. Series of experiments using ovariectomized and hypophysectomized-ovariectomized rats, in conjunction with replacement therapy of mammotropic hormones, led Dr. Turner to conclude that the physiological processes of mammogenesis, lactogenesis, and galactopoiesis were affected maximally by the synergistic actions of several hormones, with prolactin being the primary stimulator in all three phases of the sequence building to maximum lactation. However, in spite of the biochemical evidence that one molecule was responsible for both mammary development and lactation, Dr. Turner harbored the still unresolved concept of one part of the prolactin molecule having more mammogenic potency than other parts with another part having more lactogenic action.

More than the outstanding research which his group of colleagues executed while under his direction, Dr. Turner pointed

MEMORIAL TO DR. CHARLES W. TURNER

with pride to accomplishments of those he trained after they became researchers in their own right. Some of these include W.U. Gardner, W.H. McShan, R.P. Reece, J.P. Mixner, J. Meites, J.J. Trentin, C.E. Grosvenor, and D.R. Griffith.

Dr. Turner was also well-known for the several books and book chapters that he authored through the years. His books on mammary gland growth and lactation included *The Comparative Anatomy of the Mammary Glands* printed in 1939, *The Mammary Gland. 1. The Anatomy of the Udder of Cattle and Domestic Animals* printed in 1952, and *Harvesting Your Milk Crop* printed in 1962, 1969, and 1973. This excellent little book, concerning physiology of milk harvest as it relates to machine milking efficiency, has been published in several other languages including Spanish, Swedish, and Japanese.

Best known of his book chapters were those on "The Mammary Glands" in the 1934 and 1939 editions of the classic reference book *Sex and Internal Secretions*. He also wrote chapters on thyrotropic hormone and thyroidal substances which were included in the 1961 and 1969 editions of *Methods in Hormone Research*.

Many invited papers were presented by Dr. Turner over the years both in the United States and abroad including such countries as Japan, Russia, Malaysia, Indonesia, New Zealand, Australia, India, England, and Germany. Wherever and whenever he presented his talks his audiences received him with the greatest of attentiveness and respect.

Among the various honors which Dr. Turner received over the years, the two which he cherished most, and justly so, were The Borden Award in 1940 from the American Dairy Science Association and the Gamma Sigma Delta Award in 1955 from the faculty of the College of Agriculture at the University of Missouri-Columbia. The pioneering efforts of this inspiring teacher and researcher will always remain the strong foundation upon which present and future generations may build our knowledge of prolactin and its role in lactation.

Ralph R. Anderson

CONTENTS

Memorial to Dr. Charles W. Turner. ix

Historical Perspectives of Lactogenic Hormone
(Prolactin): A Summary of My Research at the
University of Missouri.   1
    Charles W. Turner

    Discussion 16
        Barnawell, Turner

The Chemistry of Prolactin 19
    U. J. Lewis

    Discussion 29
        Lewis, Mills, Parsons, Frantz, Jacobs,
        Meites, Sage

Secretion and Crinophagy in Prolactin Cells. 37
    Marilyn G. Farquhar

    Discussion 86
        Winnacker, Farquhar, Jacobs, Barnawell,
        Meites, Dellmann, Parsons

The Assay and Regulation of Prolactin in Humans. 95
    Andrew G. Frantz

    Discussion 127
        Barnawell, Frantz, Jacobs,
        Meites, Gillespie, Parsons

Evaluation of Research on Control of Prolactin
Secretion 135
    Joseph Meites

    Discussion 150
        Winnacker, Meites, Jacobs, Derby

Prolactin, The Liporegulatory Hormone. 153
    Albert H. Meier

    Discussion 170
        Fleming, Meier, McDowell, Sage

The Role of Prolactin in Mammogenesis and
Lactogenesis. 173
    Laurence S. Jacobs

    Discussion 190
        Barnawell, Jacobs, Klein, Sage

ADDITIONAL PRESENTATIONS

Inhibition of the Renal Response to Intra-
venous Prolactin by ADH 193
    G.C. Bond, J.N. Pasley, T.I. Koike
    and L. Llerena

The Effect of Adrenalectomy on the Renal
Response to Intravenous Prolactin 197
    J.N. Pasley, G.C. Bond, T.I. Koike
    and L. Llerena

    Addendum: Antidiuretic Hormone in
      Ovine Prolactin (NIH SP10). 200

The Effect of Ergocornine on Water and
Sodium Metabolism in Female Rats. 201
    T.I. Koike, G.C. Bond, J.N. Pasley
    and L. Llerena

    Discussion 204
        Mills, Bond, Jacobs, Parsons,
        Pasley, Fleming, Koike

Index. 209

HISTORICAL PERSPECTIVES OF LACTOGENIC HORMONE (PROLACTIN)

A SUMMARY OF MY RESEARCH AT THE UNIVERSITY OF MISSOURI

Charles W. Turner

Department of Dairy Husbandry
University of Missouri-Columbia
Columbia, Missouri 65201

In 1927 when I began my research at the University of Missouri, I became interested in the hormonal stimulation of the mammary gland. Early studies (Turner and Frank, 1930a, b) revealed that the daily injection of 20 rat units of the estrus-producing hormone, obtained from the urine of pregnant cows, for 30 days in castrated male rabbits and in female rabbits castrated before puberty caused growth of the duct system of the mammary glands to the same extent as seen during continued estrus in normal female rabbits. Injection of the hormone of the corpus luteum had no effect on the growth of the mammary gland when given alone, but when injected simultaneously with estrogen it induced lobule-alveolar development characteristic of pregnancy (Turner and Frank, 1931); however, lactation was not produced. The answer to this observation came in the report by Stricker and Grueter (1928) that the anterior pituitary (AP) was involved. These researchers, working in Bouin's laboratory in Strasbourg, observed that milk secretion occurred when AP extracts were injected into pseudopregnant rabbits (see also Stricker and Grueter, 1929).

In 1931, W. U. Gardner extended the findings of Stricker and Grueter. He observed that the mammary glands of mature, castrated female rabbits were stimulated to secretory activity by an alkaline extract obtained from the AP of sheep; the lactation was equal to that which occurred following parturition (Turner and Gardner, 1931). From these experiments it appeared that the stimulating substance was effective only in the activation of the secretory cells of the alveoli, and that the initiation of milk secretion was due to a definite "lactation producing" hormone secreted by the AP. Gardner also found that the lactation-stimulating substance of the AP, galactin, initiated or stimulated lactation in the rabbit, guinea pig, dog, and sow; however, the rat, mouse, and monkey did not respond to galactin. Also, involuted and immature mammary glands of the rabbit did not respond to this substance (Gardner and Turner, 1933). The galactin that was obtained from both cattle and sheep pituitaries was soluble in both dilute alkali and acids, but was insoluble in solutions that were neutral or slightly acidic. A method for the biological assay of galactin was developed. Galactin extracts were administered subcutaneously, daily for 8 days in pseudopregnant rabbits; on the 9th day the mammary glands were inspected. A rabbit unit of galactin was defined as that minimum amount of extract which would induce a plus 3 (entire mammary gland filled with milk) or a plus 4 (entire mammary gland greatly extended with milk) response.

Riddle, Bates, and Dykshorn (1933) reported on the isoelectric precipitation of the lactation-stimulating hormone from either an alkaline or acid digest of fresh or desiccated ground AP of sheep, cattle, or hogs. The extract caused crop gland growth and secretion when injected into doves and pigeons. They called the hormone "prolactin".

Working in our laboratory, W. H. McShan developed a method by which a tenfold concentration of the active principle could be effected (McShan and Turner, 1935). Using Riddle's pigeon crop gland assay, he found that the administration of 3 mg. of this material to common pigeons weighing 300-325 gms. over a period of 4 days caused the crop glands to increase from an average of 1.5 gms. to 2.7 gms. In searching for a better quantitative assay for galactin it was discovered that instead of changes in crop gland weight, the minimum proliferation of the crop gland was a more satisfactory index of galactin activity. A pigeon unit of galactin was defined as the total amount of hormone injected during a 4 day period which caused a minimum but definite proliferation of the crop gland of 50% of 20 common pigeons weighing 300 $\pm$ 40 grams (McShan and Turner, 1936).

It was discovered (Reece and Turner, 1936a) that the normal male rat AP contained an appreciable amount of the lactogenic hormone and that injection of the estrogenic hormone definitely increased its content. The pituitaries of both immature and mature female rats contained several times more galactin than male rats of similar ages (Reece and Turner, 1936b); in both sexes, as the rats matured there was an increase in the amount of pituitary galactin. Pregnant rats had a slight decrease in pituitary galactin at 12 days, when compared to normal, cycling rats, but at 21 days of pregnancy the lactogenic hormone content in the AP had returned to non-pregnant levels. Forty-eight hours postpartum the galactin in the AP was twice that in the normal, cycling female rat, but receded somewhat by 10 days postpartum (Reece and Turner,

1936b). Rats that suckled their young for 7 days after parturition had almost twice the amount of pituitary galactin as those in which the young were removed at birth (Meites and Turner, 1948b). However, immediately after a period of suckling in lactating rats there was a decrease in the galactin content of the AP (Reese and Turner, 1936c); the decrease was attributed to increased discharge of galactin from the pituitary during suckling. Reece and Turner (1937a, b) demonstrated that ligating the primary milk duct of each mammary gland in postpartum rats to prevent the removal of milk, did not prevent the decrease in pituitary lactogen following suckling; thus it was the stimulus of suckling and not the removal of milk from the mammary gland that acted to decrease the pituitary galactin. Selye, Collip, and Thomson (1934) reported that suckling also prevented involution of the mammary glands in lactating rats with ligated milk ducts. Also, Turner and Reineke (1936) demonstrated that milking only one side of the udder of lactating goats did not result in involution of the alveoli on the unmilked side.

Holst and Turner (1939a) studied the pituitary lactogen content of rabbits and guinea pigs of both sexes. They found that in the young male rabbit the pituitary lactogen content was very low and changed very little during growth and adult life, while female rabbits had a rapid increase in pituitary lactogen at sexual maturity. In the guinea pig the pituitary lactogen content of both sexes showed a marked rise with sexual maturity; males and females each had approximately the same pituitary lactogen content for each age group. In both rabbits and guinea pigs the pituitary lactogen content did not change appreciably early in pregnancy and increased only slightly during late pregnancy (Holst and Turner, 1939b); after parturition, however, distinct increases were noted in both species, with the rise in the rabbit being much higher than in the guinea pig. On the other hand, the increase occurred somewhat more slowly in the rabbit than in the guinea pig in which it reached its peak almost immediately after parturition. In both species a 3 hour suckling period resulted in a decrease in pituitary lactogen.

The lactogen content of the AP of the virgin mouse was found by Hurst and Turner (1942) to be relatively low; however, it was increased by 88% on the 10th day of pregnancy and increased an additional 63% following parturition. A peak of 201% was reached by the fifth day postpartum, after which the hormone content declined and was only slightly above the virginal level by 21 days postpartum.

Meites and Turner (1942f) examined the effect of suckling on pituitary lactogen content in rabbits after parturition. They found that rabbits nursing their young had the same pituitary lactogen content on day 2 following parturition as did rabbits that had their young removed at birth. The pituitary lactogen content of both groups was sharply elevated by day 5 after parturition, but the suckled does had substantially greater pituitary lactogen levels than the nonsuckled does. By day 10 the pituitary lactogen was declining in both groups, but the suckled rabbits still had more pituitary lactogen than the nonsuckled ones; by day 20 in the non-nursing does it had returned to antepartum levels, whereas in nursing does the pituitary lactogen was still elevated. Mammary secretion was more pronounced at all time periods in the nursing rabbits than in the non-nursing group, and in the does that were not nursed the milk secretion declined rapidly until it had ceased by day 20. These studies pointed out the importance of nursing on the continued elevation in pituitary lactogen content and lactation in postpartum rabbits.

Litter size had no effect on pituitary lactogen content in nursing rabbits (Meites, Bergman, and Turner, 1941b); rabbits whose litters had been reduced to 2 on the fifth day postpartum had the same pituitary lactogen levels as those permitted to keep litters of 5 to 11 young.

In a study to determine the specificity of lactogenic hormone in the initiation of lactation, Bergman and Turner (1940) observed that pituitary extracts rich in the thyrotropic and other hormones but containing only traces of lactogenic hormone did not possess the ability to initiate lactation; however, this fraction did have a supplementing effect on established lactation. Thus, the initiation and maintenance of lactation was due to lactogenic hormone.

Because pregnant rabbits have well developed mammary glands but low levels of pituitary lactogen and no lactation, it had been postulated that the lack of milk production during pregnancy was due to an inadequate amount of lactogenic hormone. Meites and Turner (1942c) reported that pseudopregnant rabbits, like pregnant rabbits, did not have elevated amounts of lactogen in the AP but they did have well developed mammary glands. Because lactation could be induced in pseudopregnant rabbits by the administration of lactogenic hormone (Gardner and Turner, 1933; Bergman and Turner, 1940), it was concluded that lactation did not occur in pregnant or pseudopregnant rabbits because the lactogenic hormone levels were too low. It had been speculated that the low pituitary levels of lactogen and the suppression of lactation during pregnancy may be due to some inhibitory influence of the pregnant state on the pituitary production of lactogenic hormone. To test this hypothesis, Turner and Meites (1941a) examined the pituitary lactogen levels of 20-day postpartum rabbits that were lactating and of lactating postpartum rabbits that had been rebred and were both pregnant and lactating. The rabbits that were pregnant and lactating had the same pituitary lactogen levels as the lactating postpartum rabbits, and both groups had much higher pituitary lactogen levels than pregnant, nonlactating rabbits. These findings indicated that pregnancy had no inhibitory effect on the lactogenic hormone of the pituitary.

Meites and Turner (1947c) injected small amounts of lactogenic hormone intraductally into the mammary glands of pregnant or pseudopregnant rabbits and observed the production of lactation. The intraductal injection of thyroxine, thyrotropin, or adrenal cortical hormones failed to induce lactation. These studies further strengthened the contention that normally lactation fails to occur during pregnancy because of insufficient pituitary secretion of lactogen.

The pituitaries of cattle were studied for lactogen content by Reece and Turner (1937b). They discovered a variation in pituitary lactogen with the age of the animals. Fetal pituitaries had the lowest lactogen content, while pituitaries from bulls and heifers contained more lactogen than those from calves. Pituitaries from older heifers and bulls (11 to 23 months old) had more lactogen than those of 4 to 10 month old animals. In cattle 4 to 10 months of age the heifer pituitaries contained 15% more lactogen than those of bulls of the same age. Decreased pituitary lactogen content was seen following castration in bulls, and the longer the castration period, the more the pituitary lactogen was decreased. On comparing the pituitary lactogen content of dairy cows with that of beef cows, it was found that whether pregnant or nonpregnant, lactating or dry, the dairy breeds had more pituitary lactogen than did the beef breeds.

Gomez and Turner (1936a) reported that hypophysectomy in lactating guinea pigs resulted in a complete cessation of lactation by 2-3 days, and the injection of partially purified galactin, unlike crude pituitary extracts, did not reinitiate lactation. However, the administration of galactin together with adrenal cortical hormone (eschatin) and glucose was capable of initiating or reinitiating lactation in hypophysectomized guinea pigs (Gomez and Turner, 1936b). Their findings suggested that the cessation of lactation following hypophysectomy in the guinea pig was due to the withdrawal of the lactogenic and the adrenotropic hormones, and possibly other hormones of the pituitary involved in carbohydrate metabolism.

Bergman and Turner (1937) examined the composition of milk secreted by rabbits after parturition and by pseudopregnant rabbits after the administration of lactogenic hormone. Comparison of colostrum with the "experimental" milk showed that the lactose and total solids were similar. The fat, however, was higher in content in the "experimental" milk, and the ash content was lower.

Meites, Bergman, and Turner (1941a) compared three methods of assay of international standard lactogen. All 3 methods used a standard response of 50% minimum crop gland proliferation in 20 common pigeons weighing 300 ± 40 grams. When administered subcutaneously it was found that 1 mg. of the international standard, which was equal to an international unit (I.U.), was required, while the shallow intrapectoral method required 1.25 I.U. and the intradermal (micro) method required only 1/160 I.U.

Meites and Turner (1941) described two methods for preparing postpartum human urine for the assay of lactogenic hormone. The quantitative assay of the urine of 10 lactating women during the first 2 weeks postpartum by the "micro" pigeon method, revealed a daily range of from 4.05 to 12.50 I.U. of lactogen. In 3 cases of hypogalactia less lactogenic hormone was found in the urine. The 3 patients having the greatest lactation excreted the highest average amounts of urinary lactogen. Pregnancy urine contained only 1/8 to 1/16 the amount of hormone in postpartum urine.

Ovariectomy in the female rat was found to decrease the lactogen content of the pituitary gland (Reese and Turner, 1937b). The injection of estrogen into ovariectomized rats or male rats resulted in an increase in the pituitary lactogen content; however, progestin injections into ovariectomized rats did not alter the lactogen content of the pituitary. Daily injections of estrogens into lactating rats decreased the rate of milk secretion, but did not decrease the pituitary lactogen. Lewis and Turner (1941) found that the administration of stilbestrol to mature ovariectomized rats increased the pituitary lactogen content and produced lactation in some of the rats; the degree of lactation was slight, however, compared to that occurring after parturition. The effect of estrone administration to male rabbits was studied by Meites and Turner (1942b), who found that this estrogen in doses of 50 to 500 I.U. per day for 10 days resulted in increased amounts of lactogenic hormone in the pituitary and in the blood. Meites and Turner (1942e) studied the time course of the pituitary lactogen response to estrogen. They administered estrone 0.3 mg./day to male guinea pigs for periods of 1 to 30 days. After one and 2 days of estrone treatment the lactogenic potency of the AP increased 142 and 204% respectively, and a 371% increase was seen after 5 days. No further increases were observed after 10 to 30 days of treatment. These researchers also examined the effects of large doses of diethylstilbestrol or testosterone propionate (2 mg./day) administered to lactating postpartum rats on pituitary content of lactogen; the pituitary lactogen was not decreased, but was slightly increased by large doses of these hormones, although there was some reduction in the amount of milk present in the mammary glands. From these findings they concluded that the apparent decrease in lactation which results from the administration of large doses of these hormones to some animals is probably not due to a decrease in pituitary lactogen, but that it may be due to a decrease in other pituitary hormones.

The administration of stilbestrol to virgin, nonlactating goats was found to produce copious, prolonged lactation (Lewis and Turner, 1942). Experiments by Mixner, Meites, and Turner (1944) confirmed these findings; the daily subcutaneous injection of 0.25 mg. of diethylstilbestrol was found to initiate lactation in virgin goats. These investigators also examined the effects of various doses of diethylstilbestrol on milk production in parous goats with established lactation. Daily injections of 0.1 or 0.2 mg. of diethylstilbestrol did not alter milk production; however, diethylstilbestrol in doses of 1, 2, or 4 mg. per day resulted in decreased milk production, with the largest dose producing the greatest inhibition.

Meites and Turner (1942d) found that the injection of progesterone alone had no effect on the pituitary lactogen content of male guinea pigs, while the injection of estrone alone resulted in an increased lactogen content of the AP; the simultaneous administration of various dose combinations of progesterone and estrone either prevented or attenuated the rise in pituitary lactogen that resulted from estrone alone. These findings suggested that the failure of the pituitary lactogen to increase during pregnancy when estrogen production was high was that the elevated plasma progesterone levels blocked the action of estrogens on pituitary lactogen, and thus inhibited milk secretion until after parturition. This hypothesis was tested further by the use of pregnant rabbits. It was known (Greep, 1941) that the corpora lutea would involute following hysterectomy in rabbits in advanced pregnancy and that these animals would then enter estrus. Thus, removing the uterus in pregnant rabbits should allow estrogens to act unopposed by progesterone from the corpora lutea. It was observed (Meites and Turner, 1948a) that hysterectomy in rabbits in advanced pregnancy resulted in a pronounced increase in pituitary lactogen and the initiation of lactation. Similarly, lactation occurred following hysterectomy in rats in advanced pregnancy, and the administration of progesterone to hysterectomized pregnant rats blocked the lactation (Meites and Turner, 1948a). These experiments pointed to an important role for progesterone in inhibiting lactation during pregnancy.

The adrenal steroid, deoxycorticosterone, was reported by Van Heuversvyn, Folley, and Gardner (1939) to stimulate growth of the mammary glands of castrated male mice. Turner and Meites (1941b) examined the effect of deoxycorticosterone acetate (DOCA) on pituitary lactogen content in guinea pigs of both sexes. Although DOCA produced significant increases in pituitary weights and resulted in hyperplasia of the lobules of the mammary glands, no changes in pituitary lactogen were observed. Spoor, Hartman, and Brownell (1941) reported that a material obtained from an extract of adrenal glands stimulated an increase in crop gland weight when injected into pigeons. Similar studies were performed by Hurst, Meites, and Turner (1942). Extracts of beef, hog, and rabbit adrenal glands were assayed for pigeon crop gland proliferating activity; no crop gland responses were observed for any of these materials.

The pituitary lactogen content of male and female pigeons was assayed by Hurst, Meites, and Turner (1943) by the pigeon crop assay. It was discovered that although the male pigeon aids in incubating the eggs and in feeding the squabs, both in common pigeons and in White King pigeons the pituitary of the male contained only one-half to one-third as much lactogen as the female. Meites and Turner (1947a) found that the administration of diethylstilbestrol, estrone, progesterone, or testosterone to pigeons failed to alter the pituitary weight or the pituitary lactogen content.

McQueen-Williams (1935-36) reported an increase in pituitary lactogen in thyroidectomized male rats. However, Reinecke, Bergman, and Turner (1941) were unable to find any alterations in pituitary lactogen following thyroidectomy in goats. Meites and Turner (1947b) reported that the administration of thiouracil to female rats to diminish thyroid function resulted in a decrease in pituitary lactogen content. The administration of thiouracil simultaneously with diethylstilbestrol did not inhibit the ability of this estrogen to increase pituitary lactogen. However, pretreatment with thiouracil for 14 days prior to the administration of estrone did result in a reduction in pituitary lactogen. In further studies Meites and Turner (1948b) found that thiouracil administered to lactating postpartum rats resulted in a reduction in pituitary lactogen and decreased milk secretion.

In a study to investigate the site of action of lactogenic hormone in mammary epithelial cells, Williams and Turner (1954) injected I-131-tagged lactogenic hormone intraductally into the mammary glands of rabbits at the end of pseudopregnancy. After 45 to 95 minutes, the glands were removed and the components of the cells were separated. The labeled lactogenic hormone was localized to a great extent in the particulate fraction of the mammary cells; the nuclei and supernatant portions of the cells contained little hormone. These data suggested that the action of the hormone is primarily in association with the mitochondria and microsomes of the cells. Later studies (Williams and Turner, 1955) indicated that the labeled hormone was associated with the cytoplasmic particulate nucleoprotein. These studies also suggested that the particulate lipids were not involved in the hormone association.

Turner, Yamamoto, and Ruppert (1957) examined the effects of diethylstilbestrol, thyroxine, and growth hormone on milk yield in a group of dairy heifers that had been induced to secrete milk, but whose milk yield was declining. The daily feeding of 10 mg. of diethylstilbestrol for 4 weeks arrested the normal decline in milk yield and in some animals the milk yield even showed a slight increase. The injection of thyroxine, 0.4 mg. per 100 gms. body weight for 4 to 9 weeks, was begun at the termination of the diethylstilbestrol treatment period; thyroxine administration resulted in increased milk yield in 4 heifers and had no effect in one. After thyroxine treatment, the daily injection of 50 mg. of growth hormone for 1 week resulted in a marked increase in milk yield in 5 of 8 heifers.

The rate at which pituitary lactogen was restored following nursing was studied in two strains of rats by Grosvenor and Turner (1957). In 14-day postpartum nursing rats, after 10 hours without nursing the pituitary lactogenic hormone content of Wistar rats was 30% higher than that of Sprague-Dawley rats. Following 30 minutes of nursing, the pituitary lactogen level decreased to about 66% of the pre-nursing levels in both strains of rats. By 2 1/2 hours after cessation of nursing, the pituitary lactogen had increased to about the midpoint between the pre- and post-nursing levels in both strains. By 10 hours after the cessation of the nursing period the pituitary lactogen levels still had not reached pre-nursing levels in the Sprague-Dawley rats; the Wistar rats were not studied at 10 hours post-nursing. In a later study (Grosvenor and Turner, 1958a) milk secretion in lactating rats was compared with changes in pituitary lactogenic hormone at days 2, 6, 10, 14, and 21 postpartum. The milk yield increased progressively throughout the postpartum period. Pre-nursing AP lactogen levels were highest on days 6 and 14, and the fall in pituitary lactogen concentration with nursing was also the most pronounced on these days, decreasing by 95% and 90% on days 6 and 14 respectively. By day 21 the pre-nursing pituitary lactogen levels were greatly diminished, and declined by only 4% after a period of nursing.

The possible participation of adrenergic and cholinergic pathways in the release of lactogenic hormone was examined by Grosvenor and Turner (1958b), who administered atropine or dibenamine to lactating rats. Each of these compounds blocked the ability of nursing to decrease the pituitary lactogen content. It was concluded that cholinergic and adrenergic links are involved in the neural pathways whereby suckling promotes the release of pituitary lactogen. Lactating rats anesthetized with Nembutal also failed to show any decrease in pituitary lactogen with nursing. The administration of oxytocin in a physiological dose to Nembutal-anesthetized, lactating rats also did not result in decreases in pituitary lactogen, and the administration of very large doses of oxytocin produced only a slight decline in pituitary lactogen levels. These experiments were unable to demonstrate a role for oxytocin in suckling-mediated release of pituitary lactogen.

Moon and Turner (1959) reported that the administration of reserpine to 14-day postpartum, nursing rats inhibited milk letdown during a timed nursing episode. The conclusion that reserpine inhibited oxytocin release was strengthened by the further observation that the administration of oxytocin to reserpine-treated, lactating rats resulted in a profuse letdown of milk. Reserpine also decreased the pre-nursing pituitary lactogen levels by about half, but following nursing the pituitary lactogen declined to approximately the same levels in the reserpine-treated and in the control groups.

To determine if lactogenic hormone alone could support milk secretion in rats, Grosvenor and Turner (1959a) used lactating postpartum rats that had not been nursed for 12 hours. These rats were then anesthetized with Nembutal, which served to block endogenous secretion of pituitary lactogen. After evacuating the milk by oxytocin plus suckling by the young, the rats were injected with lactogenic hormone or saline, and 12 hours later the milk was evacuated as before. The anesthetized rats receiving lactogenic hormone secreted more milk on the second nursing than did the anesthetized rats that did not receive lactogen; however, the lactogen-treated rats secreted less milk than did unanesthetized controls. These findings indicated that lactogen would promote milk secretion, but because milk secretion was not completely restored by exogenous lactogenic hormone it was suggested that other pituitary hormones may be necessary for full milk secretion. Other reports by these researchers indicated that the injection of growth hormone (Grosvenor and Turner, 1959b) or thyroxine (Grosvenor and Turner, 1959c) to lactating rats increased the milk yield. A study by von Berswordt-Wallrabe, Moon, and Turner (1960) revealed that the injection of both growth hormone and thyroxine together with lactogenic hormone in lactating rats resulted in a large increase in milk secretion. Later studies demonstrated that other hormones would also increase milk yield. Djojosoebagio and Turner (1964a) found that the daily injection of parathyroid hormone or calciferol into lactating rats increased milk yield, and the administration of parathyroid hormone together with lactogenic hormone, growth hormone, and thyroxine (Djojosoebagio and Turner, 1964b) greatly increased the milk secretion. Increased milk secretion was also observed following the administration of insulin (Kumaresan and Turner, 1965) or corticosterone (Hahn and Turner, 1966) to lactating rats; however, aldosterone administration did not alter milk secretion (Hahn and Turner, 1966).

HISTORICAL PERSPECTIVES

Studies by von Berswordt-Wallrabe and Turner (1961) examined the effect of estradiol and lactogenic hormone on placentoma formation in rats. Estradiol did not increase the incidence of placentoma formation following trauma to the uterus, and did not increase the deoxyribonucleic acid (DNA) concentration in the placentoma when compared to non-treated animals. Rats treated with lactogenic hormone had increased placentoma formation following uterine trauma (about 1/3 of the rats developed placentomas), and had increased DNA concentration in the placentomas. Because progesterone will stimulate placentoma formation, these results could be interpreted as suggesting that lactogenic hormone acted by increasing progesterone secretion and thus was luteotropic. Also, these results suggested that estradiol probably does not promote the secretion of progesterone.

A modification of the pigeon crop-sack assay for lactogenic hormone was described by Damm, Pipes, von Berswordt-Wallrabe, and Turner (1961). This modification used the uptake of injected radioactive phosphorus by the crop sack as an index of lactogenic hormone activity.

In experiments to study the effect of estrogens on milk secretion in dairy cattle, Turner, Williams, and Hindery (1963) found that the administration of estrogen to virgin heifers resulted in an increased capacity to secrete milk. In another study (Hindery and Turner, 1964) estrogen was injected into adult heifers for 2 weeks, followed by a 45 day period of milking but no estrogen treatment; a second period of estrogen treatment was then begun for 7 days. The second period of estrogen treatment resulted in a marked increase in milk yield when compared to the first period.

Kumaresan, Anderson, and Turner (1966) studied the effect of three dose levels of lactogenic hormone on milk yield in lactating rats. Lactogen was administered at 1, 2, or 3 mg. per day from days 7 to 19 of lactation, and the milk yeilds were determined on days 14, 16, 18, and 20. One mg. of lactogen significantly increased milk yields on days 18 and 20; 2 mg. increased milk yields on days 16, 18, and 20, and 3 mg. increased the milk yields on each day. Maximum stimulation occurred on day 20 with 2 or 3 mg. of lactogen; these doses increased milk yields by 88 and 82% respectively over the control yields. Lactogen at 2 or 3 mg. per day stimulated increased lactation more than any other single hormone treatment.

The studies summarized in this report have also been described in several previous reviews (Turner, 1939; Turner and Griffith, 1962; Turner, 1966).

REFERENCES

Bergman, A. J. and Turner, C. W. (1937). The composition of rabbit milk stimulated by the lactogenic hormone. J. Biol. Chem. 120, 21-27.

Bergman, A. J. and Turner, C. W. (1940). The specificity of the lactogenic hormone in the initiation of lactation. J. Dairy Sci. 23, 1229-1237.

Damm, H. C., Pipes, G. W., von Berswordt-Wallrabe, R. and Turner, C. W. (1961). Uptake of P-32 by pigeon crop-sac as index of lactogenic hormone. Proc. Soc. Exp. Biol. Med. 108, 144-146.

Djojosoebagio, S. and Turner, C. W. (1964a). Effects of parathyroid extract, dihydrotachysterol (Hytakerol) and calciferol on milk secretion in rats. Endocrinology 74, 554-558.

Djojosoebagio, S. and Turner, C. W. (1964b). Effect of a combination of lactogenic, growth, thyroid, and parathyroid hormones on lactation in rats. Proc. Soc. Exp. Biol. Med. 116, 213-215.

Gardner, W. U. and Turner, C. W. (1933). The function, assay and preparation of galactin, a lactation stimulating hormone of the anterior pituitary and an investigation of the factors responsible for the control of normal lactation. Mo. Agr. Exp. Sta. Res. Bull. 196.

Gomez, E. T. and Turner, C. W. (1936a). Effect of hypophysectomy and replacement therapy on lactation in guinea pigs. Proc. Soc. Exp. Biol. Med. 34, 404-406.

Gomez, E. T. and Turner, C. W. (1936b). Inititation and maintenance of lactation in hypophysectomized guinea pigs. Proc. Soc. Exp. Biol. Med. 35, 365-367.

Greep, R. O. (1941). Effects of hysterectomy and of estrogen treatment on volume changes in the corpora lutea of pregnant rabbits. Anat. Rec. 80, 465-477.

Grosvenor, C. E. and Turner, C. W. (1957). Release and restoration of pituitary lactogen in response to nursing stimuli in lactating rats. Proc. Soc. Exp. Biol. Med. 96, 723-725.

Grosvenor, C. E. and Turner, C. W. (1958a). Pituitary lactogenic hormone concentration and milk secretion in lactating rats. Endocrinology 63, 535-539.

Grosvenor, C. E. and Turner, C. W. (1958b). Effects of oxytocin and blocking agents upon pituitary lactogen discharge in lactating rats. Proc. Soc. Exp. Biol. Med. 97, 463-465.

Grosvenor, C. E. and Turner, C. W. (1959a). Lactogenic hormone requirements for milk secretion in intact lactating rats. Proc. Soc. Exp. Biol. Med. 101, 699-703.

Grosvenor, C. E. and Turner, C. W. (1959b). Effect of growth hormone and oxytocin upon milk yield in the lactating rat. Proc. Soc. Exp. Biol. Med. 100, 158-161.

Grosvenor, C. E. and Turner, C. W. (1959c). Thyroid hormone and lactation in the rat. Proc. Soc. Exp. Biol. Med. 100, 162-165.

HISTORICAL PERSPECTIVES

Hahn, D. W. and Turner, C. W. (1966). Effect of corticosterone and aldosterone upon milk yield in the rat. Proc. Soc. Exp. Biol. Med. 121, 1056-1058.

Hindery, G. A. and Turner, C. W. (1964). Effect of repeated injections of estrogens on milk yield of nulliparous heifers. J. Dairy Sci. 47, 1092-1095.

Holst, S. and Turner, C. W. (1939a). Lactogen content of the anterior pituitary of growing rabbits and guinea pigs. Proc. Soc. Exp. Biol. Med. 41, 198-200.

Holst, S. and Turner, C. W. (1939b). Lactogen content of pituitary of pregnant and lactating rabbits and guinea pigs. Proc. Soc. Exp. Biol. Med. 42, 479-482.

Hurst, V., Meites, J., and Turner, C. W. (1942). Assay of adrenals for lactogenic hormone. Proc. Soc. Exp. Biol. Med. 49, 592-594.

Hurst, V., Meites, J., and Turner, C. W. (1943). Lactogenic hormone content of the AP of the pigeon. Proc. Soc. Exp. Biol. Med. 53, 89-91.

Hurst, V. and Turner, C. W. (1942). Lactogenic hormone content of anterior pituitary gland of albino mouse as compared to other species. Endocrinology 31, 334-339.

Kumaresan, P., Anderson, R. R., and Turner, C. W. (1966). Effect of graded levels of lactogenic hormone upon mammary gland growth and lactation in rats. Proc. Soc. Exp. Biol. Med. 123, 581-584.

Kumaresan, P. and Turner, C. W. (1965). Effect of graded levels of insulin on lactation in the rat. Proc. Soc. Exp. Biol. Med. 119, 415-416.

Lewis, A. A. and Turner, C. W. (1941). Effect of stilbestrol on lactogenic content of pituitary and mammary glands of female rats. Proc. Soc. Exp. Biol. Med. 48, 439-443.

Lewis, A. A. and Turner, C. W. (1942). The effect of stilbestrol and anterior pituitary extract upon lactation in goats. J. Dairy Sci. 25, 895-908.

McShan, W. H. and Turner, C. W. (1935). Further purification of galactin, the lactogenic hormone, Proc. Soc. Exp. Biol. Med. 32, 1655-1656.

McShan, W. H. and Turner, C. W. (1936). Bioassay of galactin, the lactogenic hormone. Proc. Soc. Exp. Biol. Med. 34, 50-51.

McQueen-Williams, M. (1935-36). Decreased mammotropin in pituitaries of thyroidectomized (maternalized) male rats. Proc. Soc. Exp. Biol. Med. 33, 406-407.

Meites, J., Bergman, A., and Turner, C. W. (1941a). Comparison of assay methods using international standard lactogen. Endocrinology 28, 707-709.

Meites, J., Bergman, A., and Turner, C. W. (1941b). Relation of size of litter to AP lactogen content of nursing rabbits. Proc. Soc. Exp. Biol. Med. 46, 670-671.

Meites, J. and Turner, C. W. (1941). Extraction and assay of lactogenic hormone in postpartum urine. J. Clin. Endocrinol. Metab. 1, 918-923.

Meites, J. and Turner, C. W. (1942a). I. Can estrogen suppress the lactogenic hormone of the pituitary? Endocrinology 30, 711-718.

Meites, J. and Turner, C. W. (1942b). Effect of estrone on lactogen content in pituitary and blood of male rabbits. Proc. Soc. Exp. Biol. Med. 49, 190-193.

Meites, J. and Turner, C. W. (1942c). Lactogenic content of pituitaries of pseudopregnant rabbits. Proc. Soc. Exp. Biol. Med. 49, 193-194.

Meites, J. and Turner, C. W. (1942d). II. Why lactation is not initiated during pregnancy. Endocrinology 30, 719-725.

Meites, J. and Turner, C. W. (1942e). III. Can estrogen account for the precipitous increase in the lactogen content of the pituitary following parturition? Endocrinology 30, 726-733.

Meites, J. and Turner, C. W. (1942f). IV. Influence of suckling on lactogen content of pituitary of postpartum rabbits. Endocrinology 31, 340-344.

Meites, J. and Turner, C. W. (1947a). Effect of sex hormones on pituitary lactogen and crop glands of common pigeons. Proc. Soc. Exp. Biol. Med. 64, 465-468.

Meites, J. and Turner, C. W. (1947b). Effect of thiouracil and estrogen on lactogenic hormone and weight of pituitaries of rats. Proc. Soc. Exp. Biol. Med. 64, 488-492.

Meites, J. and Turner, C. W. (1947c). The induction of lactation during pregnancy in rabbits and the specificity of the lactogenic hormone. Am. J. Physiol. 150, 394-399.

Meites, J. and Turner, C. W. (1948a). Studies concerning the induction and maintenance of lactation. I. The mechanism controlling the initiation of lactation at parturition. Mo. Agr. Exp. Sta. Res. Bull. 415.

Meites, J. and Turner, C. W. (1948b). II. The normal maintenance and experimental inhibition and augmentation of lactation. Mo. Agr. Exp. Sta. Res. Bull. 416.

Mixner, J. P., Meites, J., and Turner, C. W. (1944). The stimulation and inhibition of milk secretion in goats with diethylstilbestrol. J. Dairy Sci. 27, 957-964.

Moon, R. C. and Turner, C. W. (1959). Effect of reserpine on oxytocin and lactogen discharge in lactating rats. Proc. Soc. Exp. Biol. Med. 101, 332-335.

Reece, R. P. and Turner, C. W. (1936a). Influence of estrone upon galactin content of male rat pituitaries. Proc. Soc. Exp. Biol. Med. 34, 402-403.

Reece, R. P. and Turner, C. W. (1936b). Galactin content of the rat pituitary. Proc. Soc. Exp. Biol. Med. 35, 60-62.

Reece, R. P. and Turner, C. W. (1936c). Influence of suckling upon galactin content of the rat pituitary. Proc. Soc. Exp. Biol. Med. 35, 367-368.

Reece, R. P. and Turner, C. W. (1937a). Effect of stimulus of suckling upon galactin content of the rat pituitary. Proc. Soc. Exp. Biol. Med. 35, 621-622.

Reece, R. P. and Turner, C. W. (1937b). The lactogenic and thyrotropic hormone content of the anterior lobe of the pituitary gland. Mo. Agr. Exp. Sta. Res. Bull. 266.

Reineke, E. P., Bergman, A. J., and Turner, C. W. (1941). Effect of thyroidectomy of young male goats upon certain AP hormones. Endocrinology 29, 306-312.

Riddle, O., Bates, R. W., and Dykshorn, S. W. (1933). The preparation, identification, and assay of prolactin - a hormone of the anterior pituitary. Am. J. Physiol. 105, 191-216.

Selye, H., Collip, J. B., and Thomson, D. L. (1934). Nervous and hormonal factors in lactation. Endocrinology 18, 237-248.

Spoor, H. J., Hartman, F. A., and Brownell, K. A. (1941). Cortilactin, the lactation factor of the adrenal. Am. J. Physiol. 134, 12-18.

Stricker, P. and Grueter, F. (1928). Action du lobe antérieur de l'hypophyse sur la montée laiteuse. Compt. Rend. Soc. Biol. 99, 1978-1980.

Stricker, P. and Grueter, F. (1929). Fonctions due lobe antérieur de l'hypophyse: Influence des extraits du lobe antérieur sur l'appareil génital de la lapine et sur la montée laiteuse. Presse Med. 37, 1268-1271.

Turner, C. W. (1939). Chapter XI: The mammary glands. In: *Sex and Internal Secretions* (Allen, E., ed.), pp. 740-788, Williams and Wilkins, Baltimore.

Turner, C. W. (1966). What causes high production? Story of the role of the lactogenic hormone in milk secretion. Mo. Agr. Exp. Sta. Bull. 836.

Turner, C. W. and Frank, A. H. (1930a). The effect of the estrus producing hormone on the growth of the mammary gland. Mo. Agr. Exp. Sta. Res. Bull. 145.

Turner, C. W. and Frank, A. H. (1930b). The experimental development of the mammary gland. Proc. Ann. Meeting Am. Soc. Animal Prod., p. 134. (abstract).

Turner, C. W. and Frank, A. H. (1931). The relation between the estrus producing hormone and a corpus luteum extract on the growth of the mammary gland. Science 73, 295-296.

Turner, C. W. and Gardner, W. U. (1931). The relation of the anterior pituitary hormones to the development and secretion of the mammary gland. Mo. Agr. Exp. Sta. Res. Bull. 158.

Turner, C. W. and Griffith, D. R. (1962). Possible mechanism governing release of lactogenic hormone. Proceedings XXII Internat. Cong. Physiol. Sci.; Vol. 1, Lectures and Symposia. Leiden, Sept. 10-17, 1962. (Internat. Cong. Series No. 47). pp. 740-741, Excerpta Medica, Amsterdam.

Turner, C. W. and Meites, J. (1941a). Does pregnancy suppress the lactogenic hormone of the pituitary? Endocrinology 29, 165-171.

Turner, C. W. and Meites, J. (1941b). Effect of desoxycorticosterone on pituitary and lactogen content. Proc. Soc. Exp. Biol. Med. 47, 232-234.

Turner, C. W. and Reineke, E. P. (1936). A study of the involution of the mammary gland of the goat. Mo. Agr. Exp. Sta. Res. Bull. 235.

Turner, C. W., Williams, R., and Hindery, G. A. (1963). Growth of the udders of dairy heifers as measured by milk yield and desoxyribonucleic acid. J. Dairy Sci. 46, 1390.

Turner, C. W., Yamamoto, H., and Ruppert, H. A., Jr. (1957). Endocrine factors influencing the intensity of milk secretion. A. Estrogen, thyroxine, and growth hormone. J. Dairy Sci. 40, 37-49.

Van Heuverswyn, J., Folley, S. J., and Gardner, W. U. (1939). Mammary growth in male mice receiving androgens, estrogens, and desoxycorticosterone acetate. Proc. Soc. Exp. Biol. Med. 41, 389-392.

von Berswordt-Wallrabe, R., Moon, R. C., and Turner, C. W. (1960). Effect of lactogenic hormone, growth hormone, and thyroxine in the lactating albino rat. Proc. Soc. Exp. Biol. Med. 104, 530-531.

von Berswordt-Wallrabe, R. and Turner, C. W. (1961). Influence of lactogenic hormone and estradiol benzoate upon placentoma formation in intact rats measured by total DNA. Proc. Soc. Exp. Biol. Med. 108, 212-214.

Williams, W. F. and Turner, C. W. (1954). Intracellular localization of I^{131}-tagged lactogenic hormone in mammary gland of the rabbit. Proc. Soc. Exp. Biol. Med. 85, 524-525.

Williams, W. F. and Turner, C. W. (1955). Association of I^{131}-labeled lactogenic hormone with cytoplasmic nucleoprotein of mammary gland cell. Proc. Soc. Exp. Biol. Med. 90, 531-533.

DISCUSSION AFTER DR. TURNER'S PAPER

Dr. Barnawell
   Dr. Turner, you mentioned very early studies of yours using pregnant cow urine, and it sounded as if what you found in those early studies was an FSH-LH like substance in the cow urine. Do you know of any lactogenic principle that has ever been discovered in cow urine or from any portion of the placenta?

Dr. Turner
   At that time our method of extraction of the estrogen from the cow's urine was simply to stir up the urine with oil, and then we let the oil come to the surface and that contained the hormone. But that's all we did at that time.

HISTORICAL PERSPECTIVES

Reece, R. P. and Turner, C. W. (1937a). Effect of stimulus of suckling upon galactin content of the rat pituitary. Proc. Soc. Exp. Biol. Med. 35, 621-622.

Reece, R. P. and Turner, C. W. (1937b). The lactogenic and thyrotropic hormone content of the anterior lobe of the pituitary gland. Mo. Agr. Exp. Sta. Res. Bull. 266.

Reineke, E. P., Bergman, A. J., and Turner, C. W. (1941). Effect of thyroidectomy of young male goats upon certain AP hormones. Endocrinology 29, 306-312.

Riddle, O., Bates, R. W., and Dykshorn, S. W. (1933). The preparation, identification, and assay of prolactin - a hormone of the anterior pituitary. Am. J. Physiol. 105, 191-216.

Selye, H., Collip, J. B., and Thomson, D. L. (1934). Nervous and hormonal factors in lactation. Endocrinology 18, 237-248.

Spoor, H. J., Hartman, F. A., and Brownell, K. A. (1941). Cortilactin, the lactation factor of the adrenal. Am. J. Physiol. 134, 12-18.

Stricker, P. and Grueter, F. (1928). Action du lobe antérieur de l'hypophyse sur la montée laiteuse. Compt. Rend. Soc. Biol. 99, 1978-1980.

Stricker, P. and Grueter, F. (1929). Fonctions due lobe antérieur de l'hypophyse: Influence des extraits du lobe antérieur sur l'appareil génital de la lapine et sur la montée laiteuse. Presse Med. 37, 1268-1271.

Turner, C. W. (1939). Chapter XI: The mammary glands. In: *Sex and Internal Secretions* (Allen, E., ed.), pp. 740-788, Williams and Wilkins, Baltimore.

Turner, C. W. (1966). What causes high production? Story of the role of the lactogenic hormone in milk secretion. Mo. Agr. Exp. Sta. Bull. 836.

Turner, C. W. and Frank, A. H. (1930a). The effect of the estrus producing hormone on the growth of the mammary gland. Mo. Agr. Exp. Sta. Res. Bull. 145.

Turner, C. W. and Frank, A. H. (1930b). The experimental development of the mammary gland. Proc. Ann. Meeting Am. Soc. Animal Prod., p. 134. (abstract).

Turner, C. W. and Frank, A. H. (1931). The relation between the estrus producing hormone and a corpus luteum extract on the growth of the mammary gland. Science 73, 295-296.

Turner, C. W. and Gardner, W. U. (1931). The relation of the anterior pituitary hormones to the development and secretion of the mammary gland. Mo. Agr. Exp. Sta. Res. Bull. 158.

Turner, C. W. and Griffith, D. R. (1962). Possible mechanism governing release of lactogenic hormone. Proceedings XXII Internat. Cong. Physiol. Sci.; Vol. 1, Lectures and Symposia. Leiden, Sept. 10-17, 1962. (Internat. Cong. Series No. 47). pp. 740-741, Excerpta Medica, Amsterdam.

Turner, C. W. and Meites, J. (1941a). Does pregnancy suppress the lactogenic hormone of the pituitary? Endocrinology 29, 165-171.

Turner, C. W. and Meites, J. (1941b). Effect of desoxycorticosterone on pituitary and lactogen content. Proc. Soc. Exp. Biol. Med. 47, 232-234.

Turner, C. W. and Reineke, E. P. (1936). A study of the involution of the mammary gland of the goat. Mo. Agr. Exp. Sta. Res. Bull. 235.

Turner, C. W., Williams, R., and Hindery, G. A. (1963). Growth of the udders of dairy heifers as measured by milk yield and desoxyribonucleic acid. J. Dairy Sci. 46, 1390.

Turner, C. W., Yamamoto, H., and Ruppert, H. A., Jr. (1957). Endocrine factors influencing the intensity of milk secretion. A. Estrogen, thyroxine, and growth hormone. J. Dairy Sci. 40, 37-49.

Van Heuverswyn, J., Folley, S. J., and Gardner, W. U. (1939). Mammary growth in male mice receiving androgens, estrogens, and desoxycorticosterone acetate. Proc. Soc. Exp. Biol. Med. 41, 389-392.

von Berswordt-Wallrabe, R., Moon, R. C., and Turner, C. W. (1960). Effect of lactogenic hormone, growth hormone, and thyroxine in the lactating albino rat. Proc. Soc. Exp. Biol. Med. 104, 530-531.

von Berswordt-Wallrabe, R. and Turner, C. W. (1961). Influence of lactogenic hormone and estradiol benzoate upon placentoma formation in intact rats measured by total DNA. Proc. Soc. Exp. Biol. Med. 108, 212-214.

Williams, W. F. and Turner, C. W. (1954). Intracellular localization of I^{131}-tagged lactogenic hormone in mammary gland of the rabbit. Proc. Soc. Exp. Biol. Med. 85, 524-525.

Williams, W. F. and Turner, C. W. (1955). Association of I^{131}-labeled lactogenic hormone with cytoplasmic nucleoprotein of mammary gland cell. Proc. Soc. Exp. Biol. Med. 90, 531-533.

DISCUSSION AFTER DR. TURNER'S PAPER

Dr. Barnawell

Dr. Turner, you mentioned very early studies of yours using pregnant cow urine, and it sounded as if what you found in those early studies was an FSH-LH like substance in the cow urine. Do you know of any lactogenic principle that has ever been discovered in cow urine or from any portion of the placenta?

Dr. Turner

At that time our method of extraction of the estrogen from the cow's urine was simply to stir up the urine with oil, and then we let the oil come to the surface and that contained the hormone. But that's all we did at that time.

HISTORICAL PERSPECTIVES

Reece, R. P. and Turner, C. W. (1937a). Effect of stimulus of suckling upon galactin content of the rat pituitary. Proc. Soc. Exp. Biol. Med. 35, 621-622.

Reece, R. P. and Turner, C. W. (1937b). The lactogenic and thyrotropic hormone content of the anterior lobe of the pituitary gland. Mo. Agr. Exp. Sta. Res. Bull. 266.

Reineke, E. P., Bergman, A. J., and Turner, C. W. (1941). Effect of thyroidectomy of young male goats upon certain AP hormones. Endocrinology 29, 306-312.

Riddle, O., Bates, R. W., and Dykshorn, S. W. (1933). The preparation, identification, and assay of prolactin - a hormone of the anterior pituitary. Am. J. Physiol. 105, 191-216.

Selye, H., Collip, J. B., and Thomson, D. L. (1934). Nervous and hormonal factors in lactation. Endocrinology 18, 237-248.

Spoor, H. J., Hartman, F. A., and Brownell, K. A. (1941). Cortilactin, the lactation factor of the adrenal. Am. J. Physiol. 134, 12-18.

Stricker, P. and Grueter, F. (1928). Action du lobe antérieur de l'hypophyse sur la montée laiteuse. Compt. Rend. Soc. Biol. 99, 1978-1980.

Stricker, P. and Grueter, F. (1929). Fonctions due lobe antérieur de l'hypophyse: Influence des extraits du lobe antérieur sur l'appareil génital de la lapine et sur la montée laiteuse. Presse Med. 37, 1268-1271.

Turner, C. W. (1939). Chapter XI: The mammary glands. In: *Sex and Internal Secretions* (Allen, E., ed.), pp. 740-788, Williams and Wilkins, Baltimore.

Turner, C. W. (1966). What causes high production? Story of the role of the lactogenic hormone in milk secretion. Mo. Agr. Exp. Sta. Bull. 836.

Turner, C. W. and Frank, A. H. (1930a). The effect of the estrus producing hormone on the growth of the mammary gland. Mo. Agr. Exp. Sta. Res. Bull. 145.

Turner, C. W. and Frank, A. H. (1930b). The experimental development of the mammary gland. Proc. Ann. Meeting Am. Soc. Animal Prod., p. 134. (abstract).

Turner, C. W. and Frank, A. H. (1931). The relation between the estrus producing hormone and a corpus luteum extract on the growth of the mammary gland. Science 73, 295-296.

Turner, C. W. and Gardner, W. U. (1931). The relation of the anterior pituitary hormones to the development and secretion of the mammary gland. Mo. Agr. Exp. Sta. Res. Bull. 158.

Turner, C. W. and Griffith, D. R. (1962). Possible mechanism governing release of lactogenic hormone. Proceedings XXII Internat. Cong. Physiol. Sci.; Vol. 1, Lectures and Symposia. Leiden, Sept. 10-17, 1962. (Internat. Cong. Series No. 47). pp. 740-741, Excerpta Medica, Amsterdam.

Turner, C. W. and Meiteo, J. (1941a). Does pregnancy suppress the lactogenic hormone of the pituitary? Endocrinology 29, 165-171.

Turner, C. W. and Meites, J. (1941b). Effect of desoxycorticosterone on pituitary and lactogen content. Proc. Soc. Exp. Biol. Med. 47, 232-234.

Turner, C. W. and Reineke, E. P. (1936). A study of the involution of the mammary gland of the goat. Mo. Agr. Exp. Sta. Res. Bull. 235.

Turner, C. W., Williams, R., and Hindery, G. A. (1963). Growth of the udders of dairy heifers as measured by milk yield and desoxyribonucleic acid. J. Dairy Sci. 46, 1390.

Turner, C. W., Yamamoto, H., and Ruppert, H. A., Jr. (1957). Endocrine factors influencing the intensity of milk secretion. A. Estrogen, thyroxine, and growth hormone. J. Dairy Sci. 40, 37-49.

Van Heuverswyn, J., Folley, S. J., and Gardner, W. U. (1939). Mammary growth in male mice receiving androgens, estrogens, and desoxycorticosterone acetate. Proc. Soc. Exp. Biol. Med. 41, 389-392.

von Berswordt-Wallrabe, R., Moon, R. C., and Turner, C. W. (1960). Effect of lactogenic hormone, growth hormone, and thyroxine in the lactating albino rat. Proc. Soc. Exp. Biol. Med. 104, 530-531.

von Berswordt-Wallrabe, R. and Turner, C. W. (1961). Influence of lactogenic hormone and estradiol benzoate upon placentoma formation in intact rats measured by total DNA. Proc. Soc. Exp. Biol. Med. 108, 212-214.

Williams, W. F. and Turner, C. W. (1954). Intracellular localization of I^{131}-tagged lactogenic hormone in mammary gland of the rabbit. Proc. Soc. Exp. Biol. Med. 85, 524-525.

Williams, W. F. and Turner, C. W. (1955). Association of I^{131}-labeled lactogenic hormone with cytoplasmic nucleoprotein of mammary gland cell. Proc. Soc. Exp. Biol. Med. 90, 531-533.

DISCUSSION AFTER DR. TURNER'S PAPER

Dr. Barnawell
   Dr. Turner, you mentioned very early studies of yours using pregnant cow urine, and it sounded as if what you found in those early studies was an FSH-LH like substance in the cow urine. Do you know of any lactogenic principle that has ever been discovered in cow urine or from any portion of the placenta?

Dr. Turner
   At that time our method of extraction of the estrogen from the cow's urine was simply to stir up the urine with oil, and then we let the oil come to the surface and that contained the hormone. But that's all we did at that time.

HISTORICAL PERSPECTIVES

Dr. Barnawell

Then it probably contained no FSH-LH like activity either. It's only steroids that you got out of that urine.

Dr. Turner

That's all we measured. We measured direct assay for estrogenic hormones. We don't know what else it might have contained.

CHEMISTRY OF PROLACTIN

U. J. Lewis

Scripps Clinical and Research Foundation
La Jolla, California 92037

PURIFICATION

The purification of prolactin is simplified by the strong binding of the hormone to pituitary tissue. An extreme alkaline or acidic pH is required to effectively extract prolactin and this provides a convenient way of removing a large number of serum and pituitary proteins by an initial extraction near neutrality. The first extraction can be made by homogenization of pituitary glands with 0.9% saline (Lewis, Singh, and Seavey, 1971) which is effective for glands of both mammalian and non-mammalian species, or various acidic buffers can be used (Ellis, Grindeland, Nuenke, and Callahan, 1969; Hwang, Robertson, Guyda, and Friesen, 1973). After the initial extraction, prolactin is recovered by treating the tissue with an alkaline buffer (pH 10-11), either aqueous or ethanolic (Ellis *et al.*, 1969; Lewis, Singh, and Seavey, 1972a; Hwang *et al.*, 1973), since prolactin is soluble in this concentration of organic solvent so significant purification can be achieved in a single step. Prolactin can also be extracted from pituitary tissue at acidic conditions (pH 2-3) but this method has not been used frequently. The procedure of Lyons (1937) is the best example of this type of extraction.

Although alkaline extraction permits recovery of a significant amount of prolactin from human pituitary glands, about 70% of the hormone detected by radioimmunoassay in homogenates of the glands

---

Supported by NIH Grants AM09537 and Grant BC104 from the American Cancer Society.

is not recovered. For the most part it remains in various "insoluble" fractions (Hwang et al., 1973). This may be caused by tenacious binding of the prolactin to tissue components or formation of more insoluble, high molecular weight aggregates. Another explanation may be that the radioimmunoassay gives a deceivingly high value for the amount of intact, monomeric prolactin in the gland. We have tried urea, guanidine, sodium dodecyl sulfate, and HCl-acetone to recover the "insoluble" prolactin but none was successful in yielding a purified prolactin.

The recovery of human prolactin is even lower if the pituitary glands are stored in acetone prior to extraction. We estimate that the yield is about one-tenth that obtained with fresh frozen glands. The difficulty arises only in the initial extraction of the hormone from the tissue, for as with extraction of fresh frozen glands, once prolactin is in soluble form, it remains quite soluble throughout the rest of the purification. The reason for the strong binding of prolactin to cellular constituents is not known.

The steps in the purification, subsequent to extraction, are quite straightforward (Ellis et al., 1969; Hwang et al., 1973; Lewis and Singh, 1973). Chromatography on Sephadex eliminates higher and lower molecular weight substances from the extract and provides a preparation of prolactin that is contaminated principally with growth hormone. This growth hormone, together with other components of similar molecular weights but different charges, can be removed by ion exchange chromatography. DEAE and CM celluloses accomplish the task very effectively. Using this protocol we successfully purified prolactin from eight different species and only in the case of human prolactin was there detectable amounts of growth hormone (2%-5% by radioimmunoassay). Because the isoelectric points of prolactin and human growth hormone are closer to each other than is the case in other species, the separation of the two hormones is made more difficult. Affinity chromatography effectively lowers the growth hormone contamination to less than 1% (Hwang et al., 1973).

MONITORING FRACTIONATION OF PITUITARY GLANDS

Success in isolation of prolactin, as with any substance, is dependent upon the accuracy with which a fractionation procedure can be monitored. Bioassays for prolactin are tedious and imprecise and detect all modifications of the hormone present in an extract. Radioimmunoassay requires an antiserum that reacts with the prolactin under study, and as with the bioassay, the immunological assay usually detects aggregated and other modified forms of the hormone. Knowledge of these modifications is important, of course, but in working out a purification procedure for the first time, such information can be confusing. In such a case a physicochemical procedure, disc electrophoresis, can be helpful. Here, one must first identify unaltered, monomeric prolactin as an electrophoretic component of a pituitary extract. This identification can be done by immunological or biological tests on protein extracted from the electorphroesis gel. Once the band is identified, analysis of fractions can proceed rapidly and accurately. Size and charge modifications can be disregarded and all procedures designed to isolate the one desired component. In addition, the electrophoretic method indicates whether a purification step to remove an impurity should be based on charge or size differences and gives a semiquantitative indication of the magnitude of the difference.

DEAMIDATION

The asparagine and/or glutamine residues in prolactin can deamidate to produce more acidic modifications (Graf, 1969; Lewis, Cheever, and Hopkins, 1970). This type of conversion is easily detected by disc electrophoresis at pH 10 and is characterized by appearance of faster migrating components. A banded electrophoretic pattern for "highly purified" prolactin is quite common. The deamidation occurs in aqueous alkaline buffers above pH 7.5 (Lewis et al., 1970), the rate of loss of ammonia increasing with increasing pH. The reaction also is accelerated by high ionic strength, such as used in fractionation with ammonium sulfate, and by an increase in temperature. Fortunately, it is quite easy to remove the deamidated forms from the native form by chromatography on DEAE-cellulose (Graf, 1969). If the temperature is kept near 5° and the pH close to 7, the solution of prolactin from the chromatography column will remain free of deamidated forms for at least a week.

No detailed studies have been done to evaluate the biological activity of the deamidated forms of prolactin. The limited studies that have been done indicate that desamido modifications are active but quantitative differences are not known (Ferguson and Wallace, 1961; Graf, Cseh, Nagy, and Kurcz, 1970).

The loss of ammonia during deamidation has been measured (Lewis et al., 1970). The results indicated that one mole of NH_3 was liberated during conversion of the native hormone to the first deamidated form. Because the ionization of the newly formed carboxyl group of deamidated asparagine or glutamine is suppressed at pH 4, a deamidated sample of prolactin migrates as a single, though rather broad, band when analyzed by disc electrophoresis at that pH (Lewis and Singh, 1973).

Graf et al. (1970) have found that the asparagine at position 6 in ovine prolactin is the residue that deamidates most readily. There were indications that other asparagine residues also deamidated but 70% of the first desamido form was a result of deamidation of asparagine 6. These results indicate that the electrophoretic bands of deamidated forms are mixtures of isomers, a type of heterogeneity that has been detected by isoelectric focusing (Lewis et al., 1970).

Graf, Bajusz, Patthy, Barat, and Cseh (1971) have proposed a mechanism for the alkaline deamidation of asparaginyl residues. The amide group is hydrolyzed with loss of ammonia, through formation of a succinimide ring. The ring can then be opened with alkali to produce either the α or β asparagyl form. The ease of formation of the succinimide ring is dependent upon the residue that is COOH-terminal to the asparagine. Deamidation occurs most readily if the residue is glycine because of a minimum of steric hindrance. This would explain the ease of deamidation of asparagine 6 in ovine prolactin for residue 7 is glycine. Since glutamine residues lose ammonia very slowly under alkaline conditions, the heterogeneity seen for prolactin is for the most part a result of deamidation of asparagyl residues.

AGGREGATION

In addition to the deamidated modifications, aggregated forms are frequently found in preparation of prolactin. The polymers can be detected easily by gel electrophoresis (Cheever and Lewis, 1969).

The conditions that promote association of ovine prolactin were studied by Squire, Starman, and Li (1963). Procedures that are considered to be quite mild, such as perevaporation, freezing, and lyophilization all caused formation of higher molecular weight forms. Much of this aggregated material was irreversibly polymerized. These studies indicate that care is needed to prepare prolactin that is free of the high molecular weight forms and should always be considered when interpreting data obtained with incompletely purified samples. No detailed study has been made of the biological and immunological properties of the polymeric forms. Sephadex chromatography is an effective way to remove the aggregates and the purified prolactin will remain free of the higher molecular weight forms if the solution is not frozen or lyophilized.

ENZYMIC ALTERATION

Proteinases frequently contaminate preparations of growth hormone isolated from fresh frozen pituitary glands (Singh, Seavey, Rice, Lindsey, and Lewis, 1974). Enzymic contamination of purified preparations of prolactin seems to be much less of a problem. In serial extractions of pituitary glands, prolactin is usually the last hormone to be extracted and the enzymes are probably removed before this final extraction step. That proteinases can cause difficulties is indicated by the work of Kwa, Verstraeten, and Scheidjde-Bakker (1972) where improved yields of mouse prolactin were obtained when a pancreatic trypsin inhibitor was used during isolation of the hormone from a granular fraction of the glands. Recently Watterson and Mills (1974) produced a biologically active altered form of ovine prolactin by digestion with plasmin. The cleavage appeared to have occurred in the large disulfide loop of the hormone.

CHEMICAL MODIFICATION

In contrast to growth hormone, prolactin loses crop sac stimulating activity when reduced and carbamidomethylated (Li, 1957). These results with the prolactin must be confirmed and if found to be correct, present an interesting problem. The prolactin activity of human growth hormone is not dependent upon integrity of the disulfide bridges (Bewley, Brovetto-Cruz, and Li, 1969) whereas at the present time it appears that the biological activity of prolactin is destroyed by cleavage of the disulfide bonds.

Other reactions for prolactin have been reviewed by Dixon (1964). Acetylation of prolactin with ketene or esterification of the carboxyl groups of the hormone cause a loss of crop sac stimulating activity. Conversion of the lysines to homoarginine by guanidation or nitration of the tyrosines with tetranitromethane (Ma, Brovetto-Cruz, and Li, 1970) did not alter the crop sac stimulating activity.

PHYSICOCHEMICAL PROPERTIES

Growth hormone and prolactin, besides having a high optical rotary dispersion constant (50%-60%), show a remarkable degree of conformational similarity (Aloj and Edelhoch, 1970; Bewley and Li, 1971). Fluorescence, polarization of fluorescence, absorption, optical rotation, and circular dichroism were used in these studies. Unusual stability to extremes of pH and perturbing agents, such as urea and organic solvents, were distinctive features of the configuration observed for both prolactin and growth hormone. All conformational changes produced by the agents were reversible upon removal of the perturbants by dialysis. The unusual stability of the hormonal activity of prolactin (White, Bonsnes, and Long, 1942) is in accord with these physical measurements.

The molecular weights of all prolactins studied have been close to 23,000. Prolactin of the pig, sheep, cow, horse, goat, whale, turtle, and frog have been studied. A growth hormone-prolactin-like protein from the shark also has a molecular weight near 20,000 (Lewis, Singh, Seavey, Lasker, and Pickford, 1972b).

PRIMARY STRUCTURE

The complete amino acid sequence has been reported for the prolactins of three species: ovine (Li, Dixon, Lo, Schmidt, and Pankov, 1970), porcine (Li, 1973), and bovine (Wallis, 1974).

These are shown in Figure 1. The structure of the bovine hormone is written out completely. Areas of the ovine and porcine sequences that are identical with this structure are indicated by a straight line; only positions that differ from the bovine structure are written in. Ovine and bovine prolactins differ in three places, residues 107 and 165, and an additional leucine was found at position 88 in the bovine hormone. There was an 82% homology between the ovine and porcine hormone; 162 of a total 198 residues were identical.

Portions of the structure of human prolactin have been reported by Niall, Hogan, Tregear, Segre, Hwang, and Friesen (1973). These sequences are shown in Figure 1. Included in the structure for human prolactin are tentative sequences (Seavey, Singh, Lindsey, and Lewis, 1973) determined by homology with similar tryptic peptides of the ovine hormone. These areas are enclosed in (( )). Also shown in Figure 1 is a partial sequence for whale prolactin (Seavey *et al.*, unpublished). Portions were sequenced by the dansyl-Edman procedure but those that were determined by homology are enclosed in { }. Striking homology is seen between the porcine and whale prolactins with 95% of the positions being identical. A similar degree of homology has been found for the growth hormones of these two species (Seavey *et al.*, unpublished).

From the sequence of human prolactin it can be seen that the hormone is more closely related to the prolactins of other species than to the growth hormones, including that of man. Structural similarities of the prolactins, the growth hormones and human placental lactogen have been pointed out (Sherwood, 1967; Bewley and Li, 1971; Niall, Hogan, Sauer, Rosenblum, and Greenwood, 1971; Wallis, 1971; Fellows, 1973). A limited degree of homology between prolactin and growth hormone and the glycoprotein hormones of the pituitary gland has been shown by Fellows (1973). In addition to this external homology of the hormones Niall *et al.* (1971) made the interesting observation of internal homologies in growth hormone, prolactin and placental lactogen. Four main regions within each of the hormones were found to be homologous. This led the authors to postulate that the hormones arose from a shorter primordial peptide of about 25-50 residues through two successive tandem duplications of the original structural cistron. Such a peptide probably will not be found in the vertebrates since the growth hormone of an elasmobrach, the blue shark, was found to be similar in molecular weight and structure to mammalian growth hormone (Lewis, Singh, Seavey, and Lambert, 1974). Curiously, the protein also had properties of prolactin. The only other vertebrates that can be considered more primitive than the elasmobrachs are the lamprey and hagfish, both cyclostomes, and it will be most interesting to know the chemistry of the pituitary hormones of these species. That growth hormone and prolactin may have arisen from a common ancestral protein is supported by the studies of Hayashida, Licht, and

CHEMISTRY OF PROLACTIN

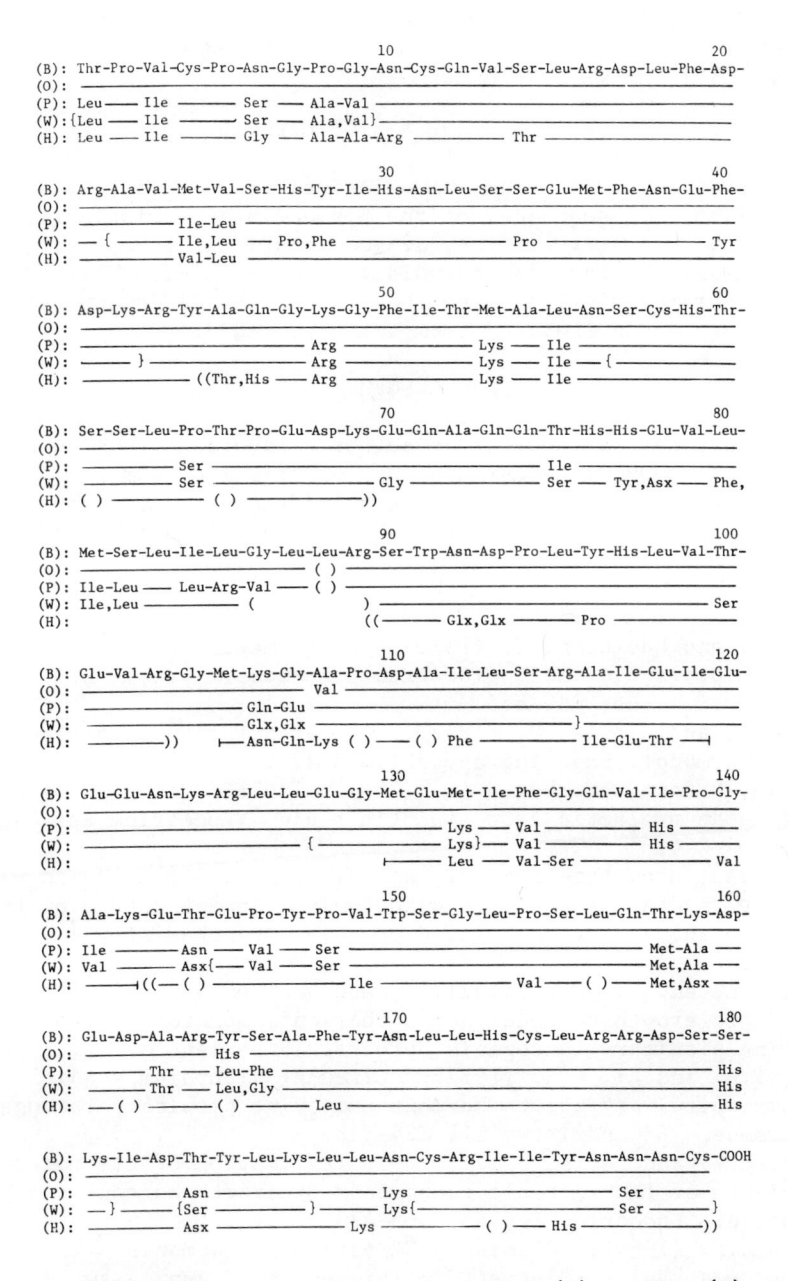

```
                        10                                              20
(B): Thr-Pro-Val-Cys-Pro-Asn-Gly-Pro-Gly-Asn-Cys-Gln-Val-Ser-Leu-Arg-Asp-Leu-Phe-Asp-
(O): ─────────────────────────────────────────────────────────────────────────────────
(P): Leu──── Ile ──────── Ser ──── Ala-Val ──────────────────────────────────────────
(W): {Leu ── Ile ──────── Ser ──── Ala,Val} ─────────────────────────────────────────
(H): Leu ─── Ile ──────── Gly ──── Ala-Ala-Arg ─────────── Thr ──────────────────────

                        30                                              40
(B): Arg-Ala-Val-Met-Val-Ser-His-Tyr-Ile-His-Asn-Leu-Ser-Ser-Glu-Met-Phe-Asn-Glu-Phe-
(O): ─────────────────────────────────────────────────────────────────────────────────
(P): ──────────── Ile-Leu ───────────────────────────────────────────────────────────
(W): ─{ ───────── Ile,Leu ──── Pro,Phe ───────────── Pro ────────────────────── Tyr
(H): ──────────── Val-Leu ───────────────────────────────────────────────────────────

                        50                                              60
(B): Asp-Lys-Arg-Tyr-Ala-Gln-Gly-Lys-Gly-Phe-Ile-Thr-Met-Ala-Leu-Asn-Ser-Cys-His-Thr-
(O): ─────────────────────────────────────────────────────────────────────────────────
(P): ────────────────────── Arg ────────── Lys ──── Ile ─────────────────────────────
(W): ─────── } ───────────── Arg ────────── Lys ──── Ile ── { ───────────────────────
(H): ──────────── ((Thr,His ── Arg ────────── Lys ──── Ile ──────────────────────────

                        70                                              80
(B): Ser-Ser-Leu-Pro-Thr-Pro-Glu-Asp-Lys-Glu-Gln-Ala-Gln-Gln-Thr-His-His-Glu-Val-Leu-
(O): ─────────────────────────────────────────────────────────────────────────────────
(P): ──────── Ser ──────────────────────────── Ile ──────────────────────────────────
(W): ──────── Ser ──────────────── Gly ─────────────── Ser ──── Tyr,Asx ──── Phe,
(H): ( ) ──────────── ( ) ─────────── ))

                        90                                              100
(B): Met-Ser-Leu-Ile-Leu-Gly-Leu-Leu-Arg-Ser-Trp-Asn-Asp-Pro-Leu-Tyr-His-Leu-Val-Thr-
(O): Ile-Leu ──────────────── ( ) ───────────────────────────────────────────────────
(P): Ile-Leu ──── Leu-Arg-Val ──── ( ) ──────────────────────────────────────────────
(W): Ile,Leu ─────────── ( ──────── ) ────────────────────────────────────────── Ser
(H): ──────────────── (( ───── Glx,Glx ───────── Pro ────────────────

                        110                                             120
(B): Glu-Val-Arg-Gly-Met-Lys-Gly-Ala-Pro-Asp-Ala-Ile-Leu-Ser-Arg-Ala-Ile-Glu-Ile-Glu-
(O): ──────────────────────────────────── Val ───────────────────────────────────────
(P): ──────────── Gln-Glu ───────────────────────────────────────────────────────────
(W): ──────────── Glx,Glx ───────────────────────────────── } ───────────────────────
(H): ─────── )) ├──Asn-Gln-Lys ( ) ──── ( ) Phe ──────────── Ile-Glu-Thr ──┤

                        130                                             140
(B): Glu-Glu-Asn-Lys-Arg-Leu-Leu-Glu-Gly-Met-Glu-Met-Ile-Phe-Gly-Gln-Val-Ile-Pro-Gly-
(O): ─────────────────────────────────────────────────────────────────────────────────
(P): ──────────────────────────────────── Lys ──── Val ───────────── His ────────────
(W): ───────────────────── { ──────── Lys} ── Val ───────────── His ─────────────────
(H): ├──────── Leu ──── Val-Ser ─────────────── Val

                        150                                             160
(B): Ala-Lys-Glu-Thr-Glu-Pro-Tyr-Pro-Val-Trp-Ser-Gly-Leu-Pro-Ser-Leu-Gln-Thr-Lys-Asp-
(O): ─────────────────────────────────────────────────────────────────────────────────
(P): Ile ──── Asn ──── Val ──── Ser ────────────────────────────────── Met-Ala
(W): Val ──────── Asx{── Val ──── Ser ──────────────────────────────── Met,Ala
(H): ─┤((── ( ) ───────────── Ile ─────────── Val ──── ( ) ── Met,Asx

                        170                                             180
(B): Glu-Asp-Ala-Arg-Tyr-Ser-Ala-Phe-Tyr-Asn-Leu-Leu-His-Cys-Leu-Arg-Arg-Asp-Ser-Ser-
(O): ──────── His ───────────────────────────────────────────────────────────────────
(P): ──────── Thr ──── Leu-Phe ─────────────────────────────────────────────── His
(W): ──────── Thr ──── Leu,Gly ─────────────────────────────────────────────── His
(H): ── ( ) ──────── ( ) ──── Leu ─────────────────────────────────────────── His

(B): Lys-Ile-Asp-Thr-Tyr-Leu-Lys-Leu-Leu-Asn-Cys-Arg-Ile-Ile-Tyr-Asn-Asn-Asn-Cys-COOH
(O): ─────────────────────────────────────────────────────────────────────────────────
(P): ──────── Asn ──────────── Lys ──────────────── Ser ────
(W): ─} ──── {Ser ────────── } ──── Lys{ ──────────────── Ser ────── }
(H): ──────── Asx ─────────── Lys ─────────── ( ) ──── His ────────────── ))
```

Figure 1. The primary structures of bovine (B), ovine (O), porcine (P), whale (W), and human prolactins. For details see text.

Nicoll (1973). Both the growth hormone and prolactin identified from amphibian pituitary glands showed immunological reactivity with antiserum to rat growth hormone.

PROLACTIN OF AMNIOTIC FLUID

The physicochemical and immunological properties, as well as a partial amino acid sequence, of the prolactin of amniotic fluid indicate that it is very similar, if not identical, to the pituitary protein (Hwang, Murray, Jacobs, Niall, and Friesen, 1974). Ben-David and Chrambach (1974) have reported on the electrophoretic behavior of prolactin isolated from amniotic fluid.

ACKNOWLEDGEMENTS

The work carried out in the author's laboratory was supported by NIH Grants AM09537 and AM16065 and Grant BC104 from the American Cancer Society. Studies with human prolactin were made possible by an award of glands from the National Pituitary Agency of NIAMDD.

REFERENCES

Aloj, S.M. and Edelhoch, H. (1970). Conformational similarity of ovine prolactin and bovine growth hormone. Proc. Natl. Acad. Sci. U.S.A. 66, 830-836.

Bates, R.W. and Riddle, O. (1935). The preparation of prolactin. J. Pharmacol. Exp. Therap. 55, 365-371.

Ben-David, M. and Chrombach, A. (1974). Isolation of isohormones of human prolactin from amniotic fluid. Endocrine Res. Comm. 1, 193-210.

Bewley, T.A., Brovetto-Cruz, J., and Li, C.H. (1969). Human pituitary growth hormone. Physicochemical investigation of the native and reduced alkylated protein. Biochemistry 8, 4701-4708.

Bewley, T.A. and Li, C.H. (1971). Sequence comparison of human pituitary growth hormone, human chorionic somatomammotropin and ovine pituitary lactogenic hormone. Experientia, 27, 1368-1371.

Bewley, T.A. and Li, C.H. (1972). Circular dichroism studies on human pituitary growth hormone and ovine pituitary lactogenic hormone. Biochemistry 11, 884-888.

Cheever, E.V. and Lewis, U.J. (1969). Estimation of the molecular weights of the multiple components of growth hormone and prolactin. Endocrinology 85, 465-473.

Dixon, H.B.F. (1964). Chemistry of pituitary hormones. In: *The Hormones*, Vol V (Pincus, G., Thimann, K.V., and Astwood, E.B., eds.), pp. 1-68, Academic Press, New York.

Ellis, S., Grindeland, R.E., Nuenke, J.M., and Callahan, P.X. (1969). Purification and properties of rat prolactin. Endocrinology 85, 886-894.

Fellows, R.E. (1973). Discussion. Recent Prog. Horm. Res. 29, 404-407.
Ferguson, K.A. and Wallace, A.L.C. (1961). Prolactin activity of human growth hormone. Nature 190, 632-633.
Graf, L. (1969) Problems of prolactin preparation and structural analysis. In: *Polypeptide Hormones*, pp. 255-262, Proceedings of the Fourth Congress of the Hungarian Society of Endocrinology and Metabolism, Hungarian Academy of Science, Budapest, Publishing House of the Hungarian Academy of Science.
Graf, L., Bajusz, S., Patthy, A., Barat, E., and Cseh, G. (1971). Revised amide location for porcine and human adrenocorticotropic hormone. Acta Biochem. Biophys, Acad. Sci. Hung. 6, 415-418.
Graf, L., Cseh, G., Magy, I., and Kurcz, M. (1970). An evidence for deamidation of prolactin monomer. Acta Biochem. Biophys. Acad. Sci. Hung. 5, 299-303.
Hayashida, T., Licht, P., and Nicoll, C.S. (1973). Amphibian pituitary growth hormone and prolactin: Immunochemical relatedness to rat growth hormone. Science 182, 169-171.
Hwang, P., Murray, J.B., Jacobs, J.W., Niall, H.D., and Friesen, H. (1974). Human amniotic fluid prolactin. Purification by affinity chromatography and amino-terminal sequence. Biochemistry 13, 2354-2358.
Hwang, T., Robertson, M., Guyda, H., and Friesen, H. (1973). The purification of human prolactin from frozen pituitary glands. J. Clin. Endocrinol. Metab. 36, 1110-1118.
Kwa, H.G., Verstraeten, A.A., and Scheidjde-Bakker, M.G.M. (1972). Isolation of prolactin from the 'granular fraction' of pituitary-tumor transplants: Improved method for the isolation of mouse and rat prolactin for radioimmunoassay. Eur. J. Cancer 8, 33-38.
Lewis, U.J., Cheever, E.V., and Hopkins, W.C. (1970). Kinetic study of the deamidation of growth hormone and prolactin. Biochem. Biophys. Acta 214, 498-508.
Lewis, U.J. and Singh, R.N.P. (1973). Recovery of prolactin from human pituitary glands. In: *Human Prolactin* (Pasteels, J.L. and Robyn, C., eds.), pp. 1-10, Proceedings of the International Symposium on Human Prolactin, Brussels, Excerpta Medica, Amsterdam.
Lewis, U.J., Singh, R.N.P., and Seavey, B.K. (1971). Human Prolactin: Isolation and some properties. Biochem. Biophys. Res. Comm. 44, 1169-1176.
Lewis, U.J., Singh, R.N.P., and Seavey, B.K. (1972a). Problems in the purification of human prolactin. In: *Prolactin and Carcinogenesis* (Boyns, A.R. and Griffiths, K., eds.), pp. 4-12, Proceedings of the Fourth Tenovus Workshop, Cardiff, Wales, Alpha Omega Alpha, Cardiff.
Lewis, U.J., Singh, R.N.P., Seavey, B.K., and Lambert, T.H. (1974). Enzymically modified human growth hormone and the diabetogenic activity of human growth hormone. In: *Advances in Human*

Growth Hormone Research (Raiti, S., Ed.), pp. 349-363., DHEW Publication No. (NIH) 74-612, U.S. Govt. Print. Off., Washington, DC.

Lewis, U.J., Singh, R.N.P., Seavey, B.K., Lasker, R., and Pickford, G.E. (1972b). Growth hormone and prolactin-like proteins of the blue sharks (*Prionace glauca*). Fishery Bull, 70, 933-939.

Li, C.H. (1957). Hormones of the anterior pituitary gland, Part II. Melanocyte-stimulating and lactogenic hormones. Adv. Protein Chem. 12, 269-317.

Li, C.H. (1973). Pituitary lactogenic hormone studies XXXIV. Amino acid sequence of the porcine hormone. J. Internatl. Res. Commu. 1, 19.

Li, C.H., Dixon, J.S., Lo, T.B., Schmidt, K.D., and Pankov, Y.A. (1970). Studies on pituitary lactogenic hormone XXX. The primary structure of the sheep hormone. Arch. Biochem. Biophys. 141, 705-737.

Lyons, W.R. (1937). Preparation and assay of mammotropic hormone. Proc. Soc. Exp. Biol. Med. 35, 645-648.

Ma, L., Brovetto-Cruz, J., and Li, C.H. (1970). Pituitary lactogenic hormone. Reaction of tetranitromethane with the ovine hormone. Biochemistry 9, 2302-2306.

Niall, H.D., Hogan, M.L., Sauer, R., Rosenblum, I.Y., and Greenwood, F.C. (1971). Sequences of pituitary and placental lactogenic and growth hormones: Evolution from a primordial peptide by gene reduplication. Proc. Natl. Acad. Sci. U.S.A. 68, 866-869.

Niall, H.D., Hogan, M.L., Tregear, G.W., Segre, G.V., Hwang, P., and Friesen, H. (1973). The chemistry of growth hormone and the lactogenic hormones. Rec. Prog. Hor. Res. 29, 387-404.

Seavey, B.K., Singh, R.N.P., Lindsey, T.T., and Lewis, U.J. (1973). Comparison of the tryptic peptides of human, procine and ovine prolactins. Gen. Comp. Endocrinol. 21, 358-367.

Sherwood, L.M. (1967). Similarities in the chemical structure of human placental lactogen and pituitary growth hormone. Proc. Natl. Acad. Sci. U.S.A. 58, 2307-2314.

Singh, R.N.P., Seavey, B.K., Rice, V.P., Lindsey, T.T., and Lewis, U.J. (1974). Modified forms of human growth hormone with increased biological activities. Endocrinology 94, 883-891.

Squire, P.G., Starman, B., and Li, C.H. (1963). Studies of pituitary lactogenic hormone XXII. Analysis of the state of aggregation of the ovine hormone by ultracentrifugation and exclusion chromatography. J. Biol. Chem. 238, 1389-1395.

Wallis, M. (1971). Structural relationships among growth hormones and prolactins. Biochem. J. 125, 54P-56P.

Wallis, M. (1974). The primary structure of bovine prolactin. Fed. Eur. Biochem. Soc. Letter 44, 205-208.

Watterson, D.M. and Mills, J.B. (1974). Effect of plasmin digestion of prolactin on biological activity. Fed. Proc. 33, 1512 (abstract).

White, A., Bonsnes, R.W., and Long, C.N.H. (1942). Prolactin. J. Biol. Chem. 143. 447-464.

DISCUSSION AFTER DR. LEWIS' PAPER

Dr. Lewis
  I think Dr. Mills should tell us about the biological activity of his plasmin digest of prolactin.

Dr. Mills
  There is not much I can add beyond what was in the two abstracts. That was Mr. Watterson's thesis work (1974a, 1974b).

Dr. Lewis
  As I remember, you can take out a portion of the prolactin and still retain biological activity.

Dr. Mills
  Yes, the major product of plasmin digestion of native prolactin does not lose biological activity. This is in the explant culture using N-acetyl lactosamine synthetase induction as an endpoint. As far as reduction of prolactin is concerned, if you limit the amount of reducing agent, you can limit the reduction to two-thirds of the disulfides. That is not to say that it is limited to two of the three. We have not proved it is that selective, but in comparable cases with growth hormone it is selective, and perhaps it is here too. You lose some but not all of the activity when you do this. If you then digest this material with plasmin, you don't know yet what the products really are; we haven't characterized those.

Dr. Lewis
  Have you tried oxidation of prolactin?

Dr. Mills
  We have done performic acid oxidation on human placental lactogen (hPL), and in our assay that product is inactive. In the same assay using casein synthesis as an endpoint, the product is reported to be active (Handwerger, Pang, Aloj, and Sherwood, 1972).

Dr. Lewis
  Human growth hormone was active after performic acid oxidation but can you oxidize prolactin with performic acid and have it active?

Dr. Mills
  We have not tested oxidized prolactin--only oxidized hPL. I don't really know what it means, if it is active in one assay and not in the other. If the assays are telling the truth and neither

of us is making a mistake, then the hormone must be binding, and there must be more than one type of response to that binding. We are looking at two different endpoints.

Dr. Parsons

During your extraction procedures, have you ever looked at the residues electronmicroscopically? In other words, what are their tissue or cellular characteristics?

Dr. Lewis

No, we have never looked at them. Maybe you can tell me whether it would still be worth looking at after we homogenize material in the high speed blender.

Dr. Parsons

Most assuredly it would, just to determine if, in fact, you have storage granules that are still intact. Another question: the physical chemical properties reported relate to materials from extracted glands. Do you have any information on whether or not some of these properties are similar to secreted hormones, as one could recover, say, from the urine?

Dr. Lewis

We have no experience with the hormone isolated from a source other than the pituitary. There isn't much prolactin in the urine, is there?

Dr. Parsons

The rat displays a physiological proteinuria. Animals bearing growth hormone and prolactin producing mammosomatotropic tumors have plasma hormone levels in the µg/ml range and appreciable quantities of these hormones in their urine as well.

Dr. Lewis

Dr. Frantz and Dr. Jacobs, have you found prolactin in the urine?

Dr. Frantz

We have looked quite carefully for prolactin in the urine and really can't find significant quantities, only trace amounts with sensitive radioimmunoassays, even after concentration of the urine by pressure dialysis. In this respect prolactin seems to resemble human growth hormone. This is unfortunate, as otherwise urine would furnish a useful index of integrated secretory activity.

Dr. Lewis

How about your lady who had 46,000 levels?

Dr. Frantz

The serum showed extremely high levels of prolactin. We did

not look at the urine.

Dr. Parsons

Apparently, then, again the human is different from the rat in that gel electrophoresis of urines from tumor-bearing animals does reveal the presence of both prolactin and growth hormone.

Finally, a comment. The homologies you're noting are certainly most interesting. We're studying these from a slightly different point of view, using immunocytochemistry. The lack of relationship between the rat prolactin and the human prolactin is most interesting to us because, by using an antiserum directed against rat prolactin, we can visualize prolactin cells in the human hypophysis very readily. Similarly, we can take advantage of a cross reactivity to growth hormone as well, and with antisera against rat growth hormone, visualize human growth hormone cells (Halmi, Parsons, Erlandsen, and Duello, 1975).

Dr. Jacobs

I have a comment and a question. The comment relates to the insoluble residue. In my laboratory we have been working with isolated secretory granules of the pig pituitary. We have evidence that there are high molecular weight forms of prolactin in highly purified secretory granules which can be converted by *beta* mercaptoethanol, but not by 6 molar guanidine, to materials that elute from sepharose columns at positions indistinguishable from monomer prolactin. In addition, we can generate immunoreactivity from these high molecular weight forms during conversion to the monomer form. Quantitative expression of this is very difficult, because at the same time the *beta* mercaptoethanol also tends to destroy the immunoreactivity of the monomer; however, the phenomenon is real. A variety of control experiments has convinced us that these polymeric forms truly exist *in vivo*, and are not an artifact of the way we handle the granules. We do not know if they have any physiologic significance. My question is, have you ever tried disulfide-active reagents on that insoluble residue at stage 1 and 2? The other question I have relates to the deamidation. You illustrated two possible pathways to *alpha* and *beta*, one of which involved the breaking of a peptide bond, the other of which did not. Do you have any insight into what determines which way that reaction goes?

Dr. Lewis

No, but it's my understanding from other proteins which do deamidate that it is the *beta* isomer which is the predominant one, and that's the one with the jog in it. This, to us, is again more reason to worry about radioreceptor assay activity of deamidated forms of these hormones, and that's why we are trying to learn to get rid of them.

Dr. Jacobs

What about the disulfide bridges?

Dr. Lewis

We have tried taking the insoluble residue that still has prolactin in it and treating it with betamercaptoethanol, but it got to be such a mess that we gave up. It was just impossible to fractionate.

Dr. Jacobs

One major difference is that we are starting with a pure preparation of secretory granules that essentially contains only growth hormone granules, prolactin granules, and their membranes.

Dr. Lewis

And I think one of the problems is, and we've noticed this with other pure preparations, especially these clip forms, that if you break the disulfide bridges they do not go back the same way and you can have dimers and trimers built up after reoxidation of the bridges. This problem isn't just with prolactin because almost all preparations of human growth hormone contain a dimer which will not dissociate with sodium dodecyl sulfate, guanidine or urea but will come apart with mercaptoethanol. One of the few exceptions we found was the radioimmunoassay quality human growth hormone distributed by the NIH which is relatively free of the dimer, but it does have other forms of growth hormone in it.

Dr. Frantz

Is the NIH preparation purified by means of some form of sephadex chromatography perhaps that might have excluded the dimer?

Dr. Lewis

I don't know how it is prepared, but I think the final step is DEAE cellulose chromatography.

Dr. Frantz

So that might leave it in, perhaps, with a charge separation.

Dr. Lewis

No, DEAE cellulose will remove the dimer. The slide shows that human growth hormone is quite heterogeneous when examined by electrophoresis in presence of sodium dodecyl sulfate. Samples from four laboratories contained three components and in addition, all but the NIH-RIA material had a fourth substance. We have designated these as 45K (dimer), 24K (24,000), 22K (22,000), and 20K (20,000 daltons). The 22K form appears to be intact growth hormone whereas 24K and 20K are enzymically altered forms. The intact growth hormone, 24K and 20K had crop sac values of 0.7, 2 and 9 IU/mg, respectively.

Dr. Meites

It has been more or less accepted for quite a number of years that human growth hormone has inherent prolactin activity, and from some of the things you have said this afternoon....

Dr Lewis
   Chadwick, I believe, was the first to report the low crop sac activity of human growth hormone a number of years ago; he reported human growth hormone with at best one international unit per milligram of prolactin activity by the crop sac method.

Dr. Meites
   So you think that when you actually get down to really pure human growth hormone....

Dr. Lewis
   That it will have no crop sac activity. And, it is interesting that these other modifications that we find in human growth hormone, these clipped forms (the 24K and the 20K) have increased crop sac activity, and these give the prolactin-like activity to the human growth hormone preparation. If you have intact monomeric human growth hormone we think that it will be essentially devoid of crop sac activity.

Dr. Meites
   If you eliminate the crop sac activity of human growth hormone, can you initiate lactation?

Dr. Lewis
   We don't know yet, but that's why I was pestering you so much about the rabbit intraductal assay. We have to find out whether our purified human growth hormone has activity in the rabbit lactogenic test.

Dr. Meites
   I don't think that would make Dr. Turner very happy, because you heard this morning about all the work done with the pigeon crop sac assay in mammalian species. If the pigeon crop sac assay was not specific for mammalian prolactin, much of the earlier work would be in the doubtful category. But there is still the possibility that it might have lactogenic activity in mammals.

Dr. Lewis
   Yes, but we do not know at this time.

Dr. Frantz
   When we have tested human growth hormone, including several highly purified NIH preparations of radioimmunoassay quality, in our mouse breast bioassay, we have found an even higher degree of lactogenic activity by this method than is usually found by the pigeon crop sac; that is, we find 50% to 80% the potency of pure ovine prolactin. It has certainly been my feeling that this is an intrinsic property of human growth hormone.

Dr. Jacobs

Pursuing this question of the lactogenic activity of human growth hormone, Jim, it is true that highly purified hGH, that is, the immunoassay grade material, is able to displace either labeled human or labeled ovine prolactin from both rabbit mammary and rabbit liver crude membrane particles, which suggests, since it is very nearly equipotent with highly purified prolactins, that this property may be an intrinsic property of the hGH molecule. It seems unlikely that this material would be 80% something other than what it is touted to be.

Dr. Lewis

Yes, I won't argue with that. For intact growth hormone to have low lactogenic activity in the rabbit, one of the contaminants will have to have exceptionally high activity. We are looking for that type of substance.

Dr. Sage

I have two comments. When rat prolactin is bioassayed on a bony fish, on the dispersal of pigment in the xanthophores of Gillichthys, it turns out to be a very abnormal prolactin in having almost no biological activity in that assay. Thus, when you sequence the rat prolactin, you should find a sequence that is not common to the growth hormones, as the mammalian growth hormones do have some activity in this assay. You may then have a localization of the biological activity. The second point is that I think the hagfish is not the ideal cyclostome to use in this work. In the lamprey pituitary it is much easier to get at the tissue, and you can separate off the rostralmost region if you wanted to, just as you could with your elasmobranch. It's a much easier material to handle from that point of view. Of course, whether there's any biologically active material is another matter.

Dr. Lewis

The only reason we have tried the hagfish is that it's quite abundant off the coast of San Diego.

Dr. Sage

And there's a very slight trace of the Gillichthys activity.

Dr. Lewis

As far as I'm aware the hormonal activity of the hagfish pituitary really has to be established by bioassay, is that right?

Dr. Sage

Yes, I would agree.

Dr. Lewis

It's still in question. But I think this is an arguing point for the value of comparative endocrinology. Growth hormone from the sturgeon is active in the rat, whereas growth hormone from teleosts is not; if we knew the amino acid sequences of these, it would help us immensely in trying to localize the active site of this hormone.

DISCUSSION REFERENCES

Halmi, N.S., Parsons, J.A., Erlandsen, S.L., and Duello T. (1975). Prolactin and growth hormone cells in the human hypophysis: A study with immunoenzyme histochemistry and differential staining. Cell and Tissue Res. 158, 497-507.

Handwerger, S., Pang, E.C., Aloj, S.M., and Sherwood, L.M. (1972). Correlations in the structure and function of human placental lactogen and human growth hormone. I. Modification of the disulfide bonds. Endocrinology 91, 721-727.

Watterson, D.M. and Mills, J.B. III (1974a). Effect of plasmin digestion of prolactin on biological activity. Fed. Proc. 33, 1512 (Abstract #1629).

Watterson, D.M. and Mills, J.B. III (1974b). Effect of reduction, alkylation and plasmin digestion of prolactin on biological activity. Proceedings of the Fifty-sixth Annual Meeting of the Endocrine Society, p. A-184 (Abstract #258).

SECRETION AND CRINOPHAGY IN PROLACTIN CELLS

Marilyn G. Farquhar

Section of Cell Biology, School of Medicine
Yale University
New Haven, Connecticut 06510

INTRODUCTION

The prolactin cell or mammotroph has been recognized as a distinct structural entity since the 1950's when it became evident that it has distinctive staining properties[1] and a distinctive fine structure. Since then we have acquired a wealth of new information on how this cell functions. It is the purpose of this presentation: (a) to review and summarize what is known about prolactin secretion and its regulation, and (b) to outline some of the still unresolved questions that remain for the future, from the perspective of a cell biologist interested in the relationship between cell structure and function.

Identification of the Prolactin Cell

It is now known that the anterior lobe of the pituitary gland contains at least five different secretory cell types --

---

[1]Differences in staining properties among acidophils were recognized as early as 1938 by Dawson and Friedgood based on staining with azocarmine. In 1946, Dawson, using the same stain, made an association between the presence of carmine-staining cells, or "carminophils", and high levels of prolactin secretion. However, the concept of the existence of a distinctive prolactin cell did not gain acceptance until later on with the introduction of additional staining methods and especially with the application of electron microscopy, which proved to be more useful in differentiating cell types.

somatotrophs, or growth cells; gonodotrophs; thyrotrophs; corticotrophs; and mammotrophs, or prolactin cells. It also contains several non-secretory cell types -- i.e., follicular cells, endothelial cells, and adventitial cells (mononuclear phagocytes). The secretory cells can be distinguished at the light microscope level by differences in staining properties of their secretory granules and at the electron microscope level by differences in the size (maximal diameter) of their granules. (See Purves, 1961, 1966; and Herlant, 1964 for a review of the light microscope literature, and Farquhar, 1969, 1971; and Pasteels, 1972 for a review of the electron microscope literature.)

The prolactin cell has been identified as a distinct entity in all mammalian species as well as in birds, amphibians and teleost fishes. Mammotrophs can be identified in the pituitaries of both males and females, but they are particularly prominent in pituitaries from pregnant and especially lactating females in which their secretory activity is at its height.

Light Microscopy: The mammotroph belongs to the "acidophils" of the classical, but now passé, light microscope terminology, in that its granules stain with acid dyes such as eosin, acid fuchsin and orange G. It can be distinguished from other acidophils, primarily the somatotrophs, by special staining procedures (e.g. azocarmine, erythrosin) and by immunocytochemical techniques (Nakane, 1970, 1975; Baker, Midgley, Gersten, and Yu, 1969; Baker, 1970; and Moriarty, 1973). The cell usually has an ovoid or polygonal shape; sometimes it is cup-shaped and shows a close association with gonadotrophs (Nakane, 1970).

Electron Microscopy: With the electron microscope the mammotrophs are the easiest to identify in the pituitary of the rat, as well as in many other species, owing to the distinctive properties of their secretory granules, which are large (500-900 nm) and very dense (Figs. 2, 3, 7, and 11-14). The identification of these cells at the electron microscope level was originally based on the examination of pituitaries from lactating (Farquhar and Rinehart, 1954; Hedinger and Farquhar, 1957) and estrogen-treated (Hymer, McShan, and Christiansen, 1961) rats. It has since been verified by immunocytochemistry (Nakane, 1970) in several species and by isolation of the granules and direct demonstration that they contain prolactin activity in the case of the rat (McShan and Hartley, 1965; Costoff and McShan, 1969) and bovine (Tesar, Koenig, and Hughes, 1969; La Bella, Krass, Fritz, Vivian, Shin, and Queen, 1971; Lemay, Labrie, and Drouin, 1974) pituitary. In the rat, the species which has been most extensively investigated, the mature granules are uniformly large, ovoid or elliptical in shape and homogeneously dense (Figs. 2, 3, 11, and 14). Immature granules which occur commonly but not exclusively in the Golgi region (Figs. 2 and 3) are smaller and more variable in size and shape, owing to the fact that they are assembled by pinching off of smaller granules from the innermost of the stacked Golgi cisternae (Fig. 5), followed by progressive aggregation of several small granules into larger, multilobulated forms (Fig. 6, see below). In males and cycling females the development of the cell's protein synthetic apparatus is modest and consists of several flattened elongated cisternae of rough endoplasmic reticulum (rough ER)[2] and a Golgi apparatus comprised of 4-5 stacked cisternae circumscribing a cytoplasmic area smaller than that of the nucleus. However, in lactating (Smith and Farquhar, 1966; Shiino, Williams, and Rennels, 1972) and especially in estrogen-treated (Hymer, McShan, and Christiansen, 1961; Smith and Farquhar, 1970; Zambrano and Deis, 1970) animals these structures become more highly developed and consist of numerous parallel rows of very elongated rough ER cisternae which underlie the cell membrane and extend around the cell perimeter (Fig. 3). Similarly the Golgi apparatus is enormous and consists of 5-8 stacked cisternae circumscribing an area comparable to or larger than that occupied by the nucleus (Figs. 14 and 16). Also, the Golgi region typically contains many images of immature or forming granules (Figs. 2, 3, and 14).

The mammotroph is most closely related in its structural organization and in its staining properties (acidophilia) to the somatotroph. This is not too surprising in view of the chemical similarities between prolactin and growth hormone in many species -- both are polypeptides consisting of about 200 amino acids and they have many areas of homology in their primary structures (Li, 1972), suggesting that the hormones, and therefore the cell types, evolved from a common ancestor. Indeed, recent work by Stratmann, Ezrin, and Sellers (1974) indicates that under appropriate conditions such as estrogen treatment, somatotrophs can shift from growth hormone secretion to prolactin secretion.

STUDIES ON SECRETION IN PROLACTIN CELLS

The prolactin cell has been a popular model for studies on pituitary secretion and its control for several reasons: (1) in contrast to other pituitary cell types which require hypothalamic factors, it can be well maintained removed from its hypothalamic influence (e.g., when transplanted to the renal capsule, grown in organ culture, or as propagated cell lines); (2) its secretory

---

[2]The abbreviations used in this paper are: DOC, deoxycholate; LRF, luteinizing hormone release factor; PIF, prolactin inhibiting factor; PRF, prolactin releasing factor; rough ER, rough endoplasmic reticulum; SDS, sodium dodecyl sulfate; TRF, thyrotrophin releasing factor.

activity can be readily manipulated under physiologic conditions, such as lactation, estrogen treatment, or removing suckling young); (3) the distinctive appearance of its granules already mentioned makes it possible to readily identify the cells *in situ* in the gland in electron micrographs; and (4) the large size and great density of the granules greatly facilitate their isolation and separation, by cell fractionation procedures, from other secretory granules and organelles present in the gland. As a result of these advantages, there have been more studies to date on the mammotroph than on any other anterior pituitary cell, and we now have more detailed information on the structure and function of this cell type than on any other in the pituitary.

Techniques Used to Study Prolactin Secretion

Even so, information concerning prolactin secretion and secretion in pituitary cells in general is more fragmentary than that on secretion of cells from other glands, particularly exocrine glands such as the liver, pancreas or parotid. Indeed the anterior pituitary has proved to be a less accessible tissue for the cell biologist to work with than many other glands. In the organs already mentioned there is a single predominating cell type, a large amount of tissue available for analysis, and an output of secretory products that can be measured in grams per day. By contrast, in the case of the pituitary the amount of tissue available is small, there are 5-6 cell types, and the output of secretory products amounts to mg or µg quantities per day. To further complicate the situation, until relatively recently with the introduction of reliable radioimmunoassays, radioreceptor assays, and assays by polyacrylamide gel electrophoresis, the only means of quantitating levels of hormone output was by bioassays, with all their inherent variables. Owing primarily to the large number of cell types and limited amounts of tissue available, cell fractionation (with the notable exception of the isolation of the secretory granules) has not been as fruitful an approach for the study of secretion in the pituitary as in the case of the other organs mentioned. What we have learned to date has come largely from morphologic or localization techniques, i.e., light microscopy, electron microscopy, autoradiography, histochemistry, enzyme cytochemistry and immunocytochemistry, which can be carried out on intact tissues, and which, with the exception of autoradiography, give essentially static information.

Systems Used to Study the Prolactin Cell

There has been a large volume of work in which mammotrophs were studied *in vivo* in intact animals and their staining properties and fine structure analyzed under varying physiologic conditions which affect prolactin secretion, such as pregnancy, lactation, or estrogen treatment. Indeed, studies on intact animals formed the bulk of the work done, including our own, until the 1960's.

Since, as already mentioned, the mammotroph can be well maintained *in vitro* and, in fact, the gland actually becomes more active when removed from the restraining influence of the hypothalamus (Meites, 1972, 1973), investigators have turned increasingly to the use of *in vitro* systems. At present a variety of such systems is available including organ culture (Tixier-Vidal and Picart, 1967; Pasteels, 1963), cultivated tissue lines (Tashjian, Bancroft, and Levine, 1971; Tashjian, Barowsky, and Jensen, 1970; Tashjian and Hoyt, 1972), hemipituitaries (Labrie, Béraud, Gauthier, and Lemay, 1971; MacLeod and Lehmeyer, 1972; Pelletier, Lemay, Béraud, and Labrie, 1972), pituitary slices or pieces (Rao, Robertson, Winnick, and Winnick, 1967; Meldolesi, Marini, and Marini, 1972; Zanini, Giannattasio, and Meldolesi, 1974), and dissociated cells (Vale, Grant, Amoss, Blackwell, and Guillemin, 1972; Hopkins and Farquhar, 1973; Leavitt, Kimmel, and Friend, 1973; Hymer, Snyder, Wilfinger, Swanson, and Davis, 1974; Hymer, 1975; Farquhar, Skutelsky, and Hopkins, 1975), and all these have been used to obtain new information on the mammotroph. We have worked with the last three systems and find that, of these, the dissociated cell system has several advantages over the others for combined structural and functional studies. Advantages and limitations of each of these systems have been discussed at length elsewhere (Farquhar, Skutelsky, and Hopkins, 1975). The main problem with hemipituitaries (or even tenths) is that the penetration of small metabolites (amino acids, hexoses) is uneven since they only penetrate the outer shell of the tissue. As a result radioautographic studies show a gradient of grain distribution with a heavy concentration of grains at the periphery of the pieces and few or no grains in the center. This problem can be circumvented by using dissociated cells. Use of dissociated cells has advantages in that (1) they have a simplified geometry, which facilitates quantitation of autoradiographic experiments, and (2) they provide a suitable starting material for attempts to separate the cell types one from the other. Hymer, Snyder, Wilfinger, Swanson, and Davis (1974) have already used such suspensions to produce cell fractions enriched in mammotrophs. If reasonably pure cell fractions could be prepared in the future, it would be possible to carry out further fractionation procedures and obtain reliable data on subcellular fractions not complicated by the presence of components of other cell types.

Proposed Scheme for Prolactin Secretion

In 1966, we proposed the scheme illustrated in Fig. 1 for the steps involved in the secretion of prolactin from the time of its synthesis on polyribosomes until its discharge from the cell.

Figure 1. Diagrammatic representation of proposed events in the secretory process of mammotrophs in the anterior pituitary of the rat. Prolactin is synthesized on ribosomes (1), segregated into the rough ER (2) and transported by small vesicles (3) to the Golgi complex where it is concentrated into granules. Small granules arising within the inner Golgi cisternae (4) aggregate (5) to form the mature secretory granule (6). During active secretion, the latter fuses with the cell membrane (7) and is discharged into the perivascular spaces by exocytosis. When secretory activity is suppressed and the cell must dispose of excess stored hormone, some granules fuse with lysosomes (7^1) and are degraded. The special innovation here is that there is a discharge option whereby the granules can either be discharged extracellularly into the perivascular spaces or be disposed of intracellularly within lysosomes by crinophagy.

CELLULAR SECRETION AND CRINOPHAGY 43

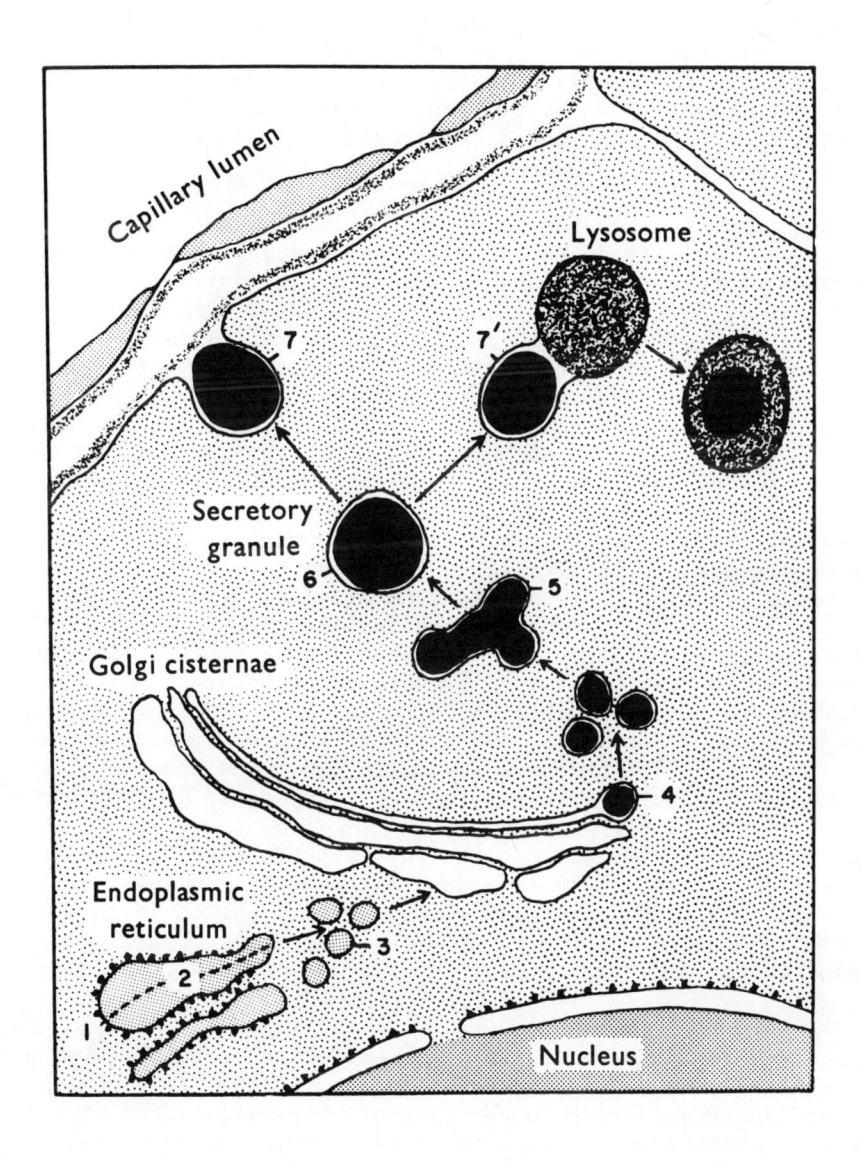

Some steps in the scheme were based on our own work as well as the work of others on the mammotroph. Others, especially the earilier steps in the process, relied heavily on the detailed, now classical, shceme worked out by Palade and co-workers (reviewed by Palade, 1966, 1975; and by Jamieson, 1972) on the exocrine pancreatic cell. This scheme has since been shown to be applicable to most, if not all, cells secreting proteins for export -- exocrine cells, endocrine cells and leukocytes (see Farquhar, 1971; and Palade, 1975).

According to this scheme prolactin is believed to be synthesized exclusively on bound polyribosomes attached to the membranes of the rough ER and immediately segregated inside the rough ER. It is then transported via small vesicles, which probably pinch off the rough ER, to the stacked cisternae of the Golgi apparatus where concentration of the secretory product takes place. Concentration occurs exclusively in the innermost cisternae along the concave surface of the Golgi stack[3], forming small (100-150 nm) secretion granules. The latter pinch off the Golgi cisternae, several fuse, and their pooled contents undergo further condensation to form the large (600-900 nm), mature secretion granules, which represent the storage form of prolactin. Upon an appropriate simulus (e.g., suckling, administration of hypothalamic extracts) these granules are discharged into the perivascular spaces surrounding the capillaries by fusion of the granule membrane with the plasma membrane -- a process usually referred to as "exocytosis."[4] Of particular interest is the fact that when the secretory activity of mammotroph is suppressed, as by removing suckling young, and the cell must dispose of excess stored hormone, some granules fuse with lysosomes and are degraded -- a process referred to as "crinophagy."

Therefore the steps involved in prolactin secretion and the intracellular sites where they take place are as follows: (1) synthesis on attached polyribosomes; (2) segregation in the rough ER; (3) transport from the rough ER to the Golgi by small vesicles located at the periphery of the Golgi apparatus; (4) concentration

---

[3] In the exocrine pancreatic cell concentration normally takes place in specialized condensing vacuoles located in the Golgi region. However, under conditions when cells are hyperstimulated *in vitro* (Jamieson and Palade, 1971b), the usual condensing vacuoles are no longer present, and concentration occurs in the Golgi cisternae.

[4] In this review the term "exocytosis," which is now in wide use among cell biologists, will be used to apply to the granule fusion and extrusion process. The term "emiocytosis," introduced some years ago by Lacy and co-workers, has also been used on a more limited basis to describe this process.

CELLULAR SECRETION AND CRINOPHAGY

within the innermost one or two Golgi cisternae; (5) aggregation and further concentration within immature granules; (6) storage within mature granules; and (7) discharge, either (a) extracellularly at the cell membrane, or (b) intracellularly into lysosomes.

The sequence is basically similar to that demonstrated for zymogens in the exocrine pancreatic cell (cf. Palade, 1966, 1975; and Jamieson, 1972) except that two main differences are seen -- one at the concentration step and the other at the discharge step. In the mammotroph, concentration of the secretory product begins in the stacked Golgi cisternae (instead of in specialized condensing vacuoles)[3] and continues in the cytoplasm in the polymorphous immature granules which are formed by fusion of small Golgi-derived packets and which are analogous to condensing vacuoles. Regarding the discharge step, it is intriguing that an option exists in the discharge operation; in the stimulated cell actively secreting prolactin the granules move toward and fuse with the cell membrane, but if secretion is stopped or slowed, crinophagy occurs, that is the granules move toward and fuse with pre-existing lysosomes.

EVIDENCE SUPPORTING THE PROLACTIN SECRETION SCHEME PROPOSED

In the intervening years since the above sequence of events was proposed, considerable new data have been generated on prolactin secretion. It is of interest that whatever new data on the mammotroph have appeared support the general scheme proposed. The pertinent data related to the steps in prolactin secretion are as follows:

(1) <u>Synthesis on attached polyribosomes</u>, and (2) <u>segregation inside the rough ER</u>: Direct evidence on these early events being virtually nonexistent in 1966, the assumptions about these steps relied heavily on morphologic observations and represented extrapolations from work done on other glands, notably the exocrine pancreas (Redman, Siekevitz, and Palade, 1966) and the liver (Redman and Sabatini, 1966). In these systems it was shown that the cells possess an extensively developed rough ER with abundant attached polysomes. By pulse-labeling and cell fractionation experiments it was demonstrated that in these glands the secretory proteins are synthesized largely, if not exclusively, on attached polysomes and segregated into the rough ER by vectorial transport of the newly synthesized polypeptide from the large ribosomal subunit through the ER membrane to the cisternal space.

As a result of this and subsequent work, the synthesis of secretory proteins on attached polysomes and segregation in rough ER cisternae have been taken as general phenomena which apply to most if not all cells (exocrine, endocrine, or leukocytes) manufacturing proteins for export (cf. Palade, 1975). The fact that the mammotroph possesses abundant rough ER cisternae (Fig. 2) which become more highly and spectacularly developed during lactation (Figs. 3 and 4) or after estrogen treatment producing "Nebenkern" - type whorls (Hymer, McShan, and Christiansen, 1961; Smith and Farquhar, 1966; Clementi and Virgilis, 1967; Pantić and Genbacev, 1972), pointed to a corresponding relationship between prolactin synthesis and the rough ER. This assumption has been validated recently by the work of Biswas and Tashjian (1974) who have isolated free and membrane-bound polysomes from prolactin-secreting GH_3 cells and obtained results effectively demonstrating that prolactin is synthesized on membrane-bound polysomes in this cultured cell line.

So far no one has carried out kinetic experiments of the type done on the other systems mentioned, but there are several pieces of evidence in keeping with two steps: First, Adiga, Hussa, and Winnick (1968) have shown that attached polyribosomes, liberated from rough microsomes or rough ER by detergent treatment, are active in prolactin biosynthesis. It is of interest that these investigators have further shown (Adiga, Hussa, Robertson, Hohl, and Winnick, 1968) that synthesis is most active with polysomes containing six to seven ribosomal units, which correlates well with the predicted polysome requirement for the synthesis of proteins with a molecular weight of 20,000. Secondly, Zanini, Giannattasio, and Meldolesi (1974) have shown prolactin to be concentrated in total rough microsome fractions prepared from pituitary homogenates, indicating that prolactin is contained within this compartment as well as in crude granule fractions.

(3) <u>Transport from the rough ER to the Golgi apparatus</u>: Here again, in 1966 no information on this step was available on the mammotroph and the assumptions regarding this operation represented direct extrapolation from the work on the pancreas (see Palade, 1966) and relied solely on suggestive morphologic findings. In the exocrine pancreatic cell, evidence had been obtained from combined radioautographic and cell fractionation experiments, indicating (a) that secretory products move from the rough ER to condensing vacuoles in the Golgi region, and (b) that they are transported via swarms of small vesicles located at the periphery of the Golgi apparatus. Since groups of vesicles of the type found in the pancreas were present in abundance at the periphery of the Golgi apparatus in mammotrophs from lactating animals (Fig. 3), a similar transport sequence was envisaged for the prolactin cell.

At present, cell fractionation data is still lacking on the mammotroph, but there is now direct evidence obtained from autoradiography of the prolactin cell, indicating that the direction of movement of the secretory product is from rough ER to Golgi cisternae to granules. Tixier-Vidal and Picart (1967) carried out radioautography on prolactin cells of the duck pituitary in organ culture and showed that after a ^{3}H-leucine pulse the grains appeared first over the rough ER, later (after 30 min.-1 hr.) over the Golgi cisternae and still later (after 2-4 hrs.) over secretory granules. The author has recently carried out a similar radioautographic analysis of prolactin cells in dissociated cell suspensions prepared from pituitaries of estrogen-treated female rats. The results, shown in Figs. 12-17, are basically, similar, as far as direction of movement of the secretory product is concerned, to those obtained in the duck pituitary and show that the radioautographic grains are initially diffusely distributed, suggesting their association with the rough ER (Fig. 12). After 20 min. to 1 hr. they are found predominantly over forming (Fig. 13) and aggregating (Figs. 14-15) granules in the Golgi region, and later (after 2-3 hrs.) are concentrated over mature secretory granules (Figs. 16 and 17). Labrie, Pelletier, Lemay, Borgeat, Barden, Dupont, Savary, Côté, and Boucher, 1973) have reported similar radioautographic findings on mammotrophs from pituitary slices.

As mentioned, the transport step by which the secretory proteins are ferried from one cell compartment (rough ER) to the other (condensing vacuoles or Golgi cisternae) is apparently accomplished by shuttling vesicles. As such it clearly involves membrane fission and fusion -- i.e., pinching off of the vesicles from rough ER and their fusion with Golgi elements. In the pancreas this process was shown (Jamieson and Palade, 1967a, b) to be dependent on the availability of metabolic energy and inhibited by inhibitors of oxidative phosphorylation, but to be independent of protein synthesis. The recent results of Labrie, Pelletier, Lemay, Borgeat, Varden, Dupont, Savary, Côté, and Boucher (1973) suggest that such is also the case for the prolactin cell.

(4) <u>Concentration in the stacked Golgi cisternae</u>, and (5) <u>aggregation of small granules</u>: The evidence for these processes is morphologic since these steps can be visualized by electron microscopy (Smith and Farquhar, 1966). Within the rough ER and the Golgi cisternae the secretory product apparently exists in dilute solution with a low electron density. Dense lumps of secretory material of high density, equivalent to that of the mature secretion granules, are first seen in the innermost cisternae along the concave face of the Golgi stack (Fig. 5). The hormone apparently remains in this dense, insoluble form until its discharge from the cell or into lysosomes. The appearance of dense secretory granule material initially in the innermost Golgi cisternae indicates that concentration must take place there.

Both the increased density of the content together with the increased number of radioautographic grains associated with aggregating granules (Figs. 13-15) constitute evidence that concentration is occurring. The fact that such concentration can take place in a continuous compartment suggests that some mechanism must exist for insolubilizing the prolactin at this site. The insoluble, non-fluid nature of the secretory material is further indicated by the polymorphous shapes of the aggregating granules as well as the fact that the content retains its characteristic form for a time after discharge from the cell or into lysosomes (see below). Recent work by Zanini and Giannattasio (1974) and Giannattasio, Zanini, and Meldolesi (1975), which is discussed below, on isolated prolactin granules indicates that indeed, in the electron-dense form, the granule contents are remarkably stable.

Regarding concentration, at present nothing is known concerning that nature of the concentration mechanism or what alterations the secretory product undergoes in this location. Cytochemical studies carried out on the mammotroph (Smith and Farquhar, 1966, 1970) indicate that several enzymes -- i.e., nucleoside diphosphatases and acid phosphatase -- are more concentrated in the inner Golgi cisternae and around forming (immature) granules than in the remaining cisternae, suggesting that the activities demonstrated have some connection with the concentration and packaging process. In the exocrine pancreatic cell it has been shown that concentration, which, as already indicated, normally takes place in condensing vacuoles instead of Golgi cisternae, is not dependent on a supply of energy and is not accomplished by ion pumps (Jamieson and Palade, 1971a). It has been postulated to be accomplished by ionic interactions between a sulfated polyanion and pancreatic secretory proteins, forming large aggregates (Palade, 1975). However, the validity of this hypothesis and its applicability to concentration of secretory proteins in other cell types, including the mammotroph, remain to be established.

From the general standpoint it is worth noting that the fact that concentration is restricted to the innermost cisternae along the concave (trans) Golgi surface indicated that here as well as in many other systems (cf. Farquhar, 1971), specialization exists with this organelle.

(6) <u>Storage in mature secretion granules</u>: Prolactin is stored until needed in secretory granules which vary somewhat in size (500-900 A) according to how many of the Golgi-derived small packets have merged and pooled their contents. In the lactating animal (Fig. 3) under continuous stimulation to discharge synthesized hormone, relatively few large granules accumulate.

Apparently the aggregation step as well as the storage step is rushed, so that fewer small granules merge, and the granules do not reach their maximal size. With removal of the suckling young and thus removal of the discharge stimulus, aggregation and discharge apparently are not so rushed, so that more small granules merge, and the size of the resulting granules which accumulate in the cytoplasm is correspondingly larger.

The storage of prolactin in secretory granules has been unequivocally demonstrated by isolation and analysis of the granule contents and by immunocytochemistry carried out at the electron microscope level (Nakane, 1970; Parsons and Erlandsen, 1974). Location of hormone in the granules was orginally demonstrated in the rat by the persistent and heroic efforts of McShan and his students (McShan and Hartley, 1965; Costoff and McShan, 1969) who succeeded in isolating the 600-900 nm granules from pituitary homogenates by a combination of differential centrifugation and filtration techniques, and in demonstrating, by bioassay, localization of prolactin activity within the granules. Similar results were subsequently obtained by Kwa, Van der Gugten, and Ver hofstad (1969) on rat prolactin granules isolated from pituitaries of normal females or from pituitary tumor transplants, and by Zanini and Giannattasio (1974) and Giannattasio, Zanini, and Meldolesi (1975) on rat prolactin granules isolated from normal females. Secretory granules, measuring 300-600 nm, bearing radioimmunoassayable prolactin and growth hormone activity have also been isolated from the bovine pituitary (Tesar, Koenig, and Hughes, 1969; Labella, Krass, Fritz, Vivian, Shin, and Queen, 1971; Lemay, Labrie, and Drouin, 1974).

Several of the above mentioned workers have further analyzed the granules and their contents in order to determine (a) in what form prolactin is stored; (b) what other substances (precursors, carriers) may be present in addition to prolactin; and (c) the relative stability of both the membrane and the contents. The information on these topics is incomplete, differs somewhat in the two species (rat vs. beef) and can be summarized as follows: Prolactin granules and growth hormone granules are more stable in both species than secretory granules from glycoprotein-producing cells. Zanini and Giannattasio (1974) and Giannattasio, Zanini, and Meldolesi (1975) have shown that the contents of rat prolactin granules have unusual stability in that the membrane can be selectively stripped away using large conecntrations of detergents (DOC or Lubrol Px) leaving unsolubilized lumps of granule core material. The latter succumbs finally to acid pH, urea (2.5 mM) or SDS (1%). No insights were obtained on the mechanism of this unusual stability, but both EDTA and divalent cations were without effect, suggesting that it does not rely on ionic interactions involving Ca^{2+} bridges. As far as the content is concerned, these workers further showed by SDS gel analysis that prolactin constitutes the predominant polypeptide present and that a few other proteins, as yet uncharacterized, are present in very small amounts.

Observations on bovine prolactin granules parallel in some respects those on rat granules and differ in other respects. The findings are parallel in the sense that work by LaBella, Krass, Fritz, Vivian, Shin, and Queen (1971) suggests that the hormone is stored in aggregate form with no precursors or carrier proteins evident. In contrast to rat prolactin granules, Lemay, Labrie, and Drouin (1974) have shown that bovine granules are stabilized by Ca^{2+}, Mg^{2+}, and ATP. However, in the latter case the authors were dealing with pooled large granule fractions containing both growth hormone and prolactin.

As previously mentioned, both nucleoside diphosphatase activity and acid phosphatase activity were demonstrated by electron microscope cytochemistry (Smith and Farquhar, 1966, 1970) around forming and mature prolactin granules in the rat. The fact that the amount of demonstrable activity parallels secretion led to the suggestion that it might be associated with the concentration of and/or discharge of secretory products. Recently, Poirier, De Lean, Pelletier, Lemay, and Labrie (1974) have reported the presence of Ca^{2+}- and Mg^{2+}- dependent ATPase activities in granule fractions from bovine pituitary containing both prolactin and growth hormone, and have suggested that these enzyme activities may play a role in the formation and the stability of prolactin and growth hormone granules. Whether or not the same or different phosphatases are demonstrated in the two different species cannot be determined at this time, and the precise roles of both enzyme activities in the secretory process remain unknown.

(7A) <u>Discharge of granules extracellularly by exocytosis</u>: The evidence for discharge of prolactin granules by membrane fusion or exocytosis is morphologic (Fig. 7). Electron microscopic images of exocytosis in several types of pituitary cells were seen as early as 1961 (Farquhar, 1961 a, b) and were first shown in mammotrophs by Sano (1962) in the mouse and by Pasteels (1963) in the rat. The association between increased release of prolactin and increased exocytosis was first made by Pasteels (1963) who showed that within 15 min. after initiation of suckling, which stimulated prolactin release, increased numbers of granule fusion (exocytosis) images were seen in mammotrophs of lactating mothers. This observation has been amply confirmed by others (Farquhar, 1969, 1971; Shiino, Williams, and Rennels, 1972). Pelletier, Lemay, Béraud, and Labrie (1972) have similarly demonstrated increased numbers of granule discharge images in prolactin cells from pituitary slices incubated *in vitro* with dibutyryl cyclic AMP, which stimulates prolactin secretion.

During exocytosis the membrane of the granule apparently fuses selectively with that portion of the plasma membrane facing the capillary basement membrane (Farquhar, 1961a, 1971; Pelletier, Peillon, and Vila-Porcile, 1971) and becomes incorporated into it. The content of the granule retains its density and the core remains visible in close proximity to the plasma membrane for a time -- usually as long as the pockets created by the fusions are still recognizable (Fig. 7). Presumably it is rapidly solubilized in the environment of the connective tissue space and disappears from view, since granule cores are not seen floating around in the perivascular connective tissue spaces (Farquhar, 1961b). In its soluble form the hormone is presumably free to diffuse through the remaining barriers (parenchymal cell basement membrane, connective tissue spaces, endothelial basement membrane, and fenestrae of the endothelium) to reach the circulating plasma. From the work of Clementi and Palade (1969) on intestinal capillaries and Pelletier and Puviani (1974) on pituitary capillaries, we know that proteins with molecular weights of up to 40,000, (i.e., horsradish peroxidase) have no difficulty traversing the same sequence of barriers; hence prolactin as well as other pituitary hormones, all of which have molecular weights of 20-28,000, should have no difficulty traversing the same barriers in the reverse direction.

Regarding the biochemical mechanisms for exocytosis, the situation is not clear. It is clear that the adenylate cyclase system and divalent cations play an important role in the control of hormone release from mammotrophs (Lemay and Labrie, 1972; Nagasawa and Yanai, 1972) as well as from other pituitary cells since cyclic AMP (Lemaire, Pelletier, and Labrie, 1971; Nagasawa and Yanai, 1972) and Ca++ (Parsons, 1970; MacLeod and Lehmeyer, 1972) stimulate prolactin release. The existence of a c-AMP dependent protein kinase was reported in bovine pituitary tissue by Labrie and co-workers (Labrie, Lemaire, and Courte, 1971; Lemaire, Pelletier, and Labrie, 1971) who have further demonstrated that both secretory granule proteins (Labrie, Lamaire, Poirier, Pelletier, and Boucher, 1971) and plasma membrane proteins (Lemay, Deschenes, Lemaire, Pourier, Poulin, and Labrie, 1974) can be phosphorylated *in vitro* by an endogenous protein kinase. They have suggested that release depends on the same general mechanism proposed for other tissues: -- i.e., activation of adenylate cyclase activity which raises the level of intracellular cyclic AMP which then binds to the regulatory moiety of an inactive protein kinase complex in the cytosol. This results in the release of a catalytic subunit and its subsequent binding to, and phosphorylation of a wide variety of substrates, some of which are in soluble form and other in the granule membranes or the plasma membrane. Whether or not this is the correct scheme remains to be determined. It also remains to be determined how other factors mentioned, such as ions, and certain structural elements, such as microtubules and microfilaments, are involved in this process.

Microtubules have been implicated in exocytosis in mammotrophs (Labrie, Gauthier, Pelletier, Borgeat, Lemay, and Gouge, 1973; Gautvik and Tashjian, 1973). As in other cells, this assumption is based on the fact that agents such as colchincine and deuterium oxide which interact with microtubule proteins inhibit release of prolactin. However, at present the situation is confused because no special association of microtubules with either secretory granules or plasma membranes has been noted in mammotrophs (Farquhar, 1971; Pelletier and Bornstein, 1972; MacLeod, Lehmeyer, and Bruni, 1973), and because in addition to its binding to microtubules, cholchicine is known to bind to membranes (Stadler and Franke, 1974) and to inhibit several transport systems in the plasma membrane (Wilson, Banburg, Mizel, Grisham, and Creswell, 1973).

In endocrine systems the question is frequently asked if exocytosis is the only or even the main mechanism for release of pituitary hormones. To this one can answer that although alternative mechanisms have been proposed, so far exocytosis is the only mechanism for discharge of macromolecular secretory products (cf. Farquhar, 1971; Farquhar, Skutelsky, and Hopkins, 1975; Palade, 1975).

(7B) Discharge of hormones intracellularly into lysosomes: Evidnece for fusion of secretion granules with lysosomes or "crinophagy" is morphologic and cytochemical (Smith and Farquhar, 1966; Farquhar, 1969) and was based on the examination of mammotrophs of lactating rats at various intervals after removal of the suckling young, a situation in which prolactin secretion is dramatically suppressed. In these circumstances the dense content of secretory granules was frequently seen within lysosomes, and occasionally images could be found of granules fusing with lysosomes. When the process was at its height (24-48 hr. after removing suckling young), virtually every low power field was seen to contain one or more lysosomes with a secretory granule inside it (see Figs. 8-10). The identification of the granule-containing bodies as lysosomes was verified by carrying out cytochemical tests for lysosomal enzymes (acid phosphatase and aryl sulfatase) (Smith and Farquhar, 1966, Farquhar, 1969).

In retrospect it is clear that the discovery of the existence of crinophagy in mammotrophs was facilitated by the great stability of the secretory granule contents of these cells which instead of solubilizing and disappearing from view, remained insoluble and therefore visible for an undefined time after their incorporation into lysosomes. Although the occurrence of crinophagy has been verified in other pituitary cell types (Farquhar, 1969) it is much more difficult to study due to the greater instability of the granule contents which solubilize and disappear from view upon fusion and pooling of contents of the two organelles (secretory granules and lysosomes).

Once the granules have been taken up into lysosomes their fate, like other organelles and macromolecules incorporated into these organelles, is presumably to undergo digestion down to the level of their constituent amino acids which can then be reutilized. Work by Ellis and co-workers (Ellis, 1960; McDonald, Callahan, Ellis, and Smith, 1971) has shown that anterior pituitary lysosomes, like other lysosomes, contain aminopeptidases and dipeptidyl aminopeptidases capable of splitting prolactin and other pituitary hormones down to the level of amino acids and dipeptides. The latter can then diffuse through the lysosomal membrane to reach the cytoplasmic matrix. In the case of prolactin and growth hormone, 75-100% of the biological activity of the hormone is lost by cleavage of only seven peptide bonds, which is carried out by a lysosomal acid proteinase.

Because crinophagy was enhanced under circumstances when prolactin secretion was suppressed, it was postulated that this phenomenon represents a mechanism for dealing with over-production of hormone. However, it should be stressed that crinophagy also occurs, though at a lower level, in normal animals. Its occurrence in mammotrophs has been verified by others (Vila-Porcile, Olivier, and Racadot, 1973). Observations by Vila-Porcile, Olivier, and Racadot (1973) suggest further that if lysosomes of prolactin cells become overloaded they may discharge their residues by exocytosis into the extracellular spaces where they can presumably be disposed of by mononuclear phagocytes. Hence the process of crinophagy provides a mechanism whereby pituitary cells and certain other endocrine cells (Farquhar, 1969) can adjust to fluctuations in secretory activity and take care of over-production of hormone by incorporating it into lysosomes where it can be degraded. The degradation products, which are released into the cell sol, can then be reutilized.

REGULATION OF PROLACTIN SECRETION

In regard to control mechanisms a number of agents have been defined which affect prolactin secretion, including hypothalamic releasing and inhibiting hormones, estrogen, thyroxine, catecholamines, and certain drugs (ergots and barbiturates). The effects of these agents have been discussed already by Dr. Meites in his article in this volume, have been recently reviewed elsewhere (Meites, 1972, 1973; Tolis and Friesen, 1974) and hence will not be dealt with in detail here. However, no description of pituitary secretion would be complete without at least mentioning what is known about cellular sites of localization of these controls, in terms of the various events in the secretory process. As pointed out by Dr. Meites, there is considerable evidence for the presence of both a prolactin release-inhibiting factor (PIF) and a prolactin-releasing factor (PRF) (Meites, 1973), and it is apparently the balance in the activity of these two hormones which determines the amount of prolactin released into the circulation. In addition, TRF has been shown to stimulate prolactin release both *in vivo* (Jacobs, Snyder, Wilber, Utiger, and Daughaday, 1971; Bowers, Friesen, Hwang, Guyda, and Folkers, 1971) and *in vitro* (Tashjian, Bancroft, and Levine, 1971; Vale, Blackwell, Grant, and Guillemin, 1973). There is no direct evidence available on the sites of action of the prolactin releasing and inhibiting factors since these two hormones have been identified, but not yet purified and synthesized (Guillemin and Burgus, 1972; Schally, Arimura, and Kastin, 1973; Grant and Vale, 1974). However, in the case of several hypothalamic hormones which have been purified, such as TRF and LRF, it is clear that they have a dual action on both synthesis and release of pituitary hormones (see Labrie, Pelletier, Lemay, Borgeat, Barden, Dupont, Savary, Côté, and Boucher, 1973; Peterson and Guillemin, 1974). The effect on release is evident within minutes and is seen as a stimulation (or suppression) of exocytosis (Couch, Arimura, Schally, Saito, and Sawano, 1969; Shiino, Arimura, Schally, and Rennels, 1972; Shiino, Williams, and Rennels, 1973; Moguilevsky, Cuerdo-Rocha, Christot, and Zambrano, 1973). The effect on synthesis is evident only after a few hours and is apparently caused by events at the ribosomal level (Labrie *et al.*, 1973) where translation of prolactin messenger RNA is presumably affected. Both effects are apparently mediated by cyclic AMP and, as in the case of other peptide hormones (Cuatrecasas, 1972), are presumed to be initiated by binding to the plasma membrane (Labrie, Barden, Poirier, and DeLean, 1972; Grant, Vale, and Guillemin, 1972; Wilber and Seibel, 1973; Goudji, Tixier-Vidal, Morin, Pradelles, Morgat, Fromageot, and Kerdelheu, 1973; Hinkle, Woroch, and Tashjian, 1974). However, binding to other cell constituents cannot be ruled out (Stumpf, Sar, and Keefer, 1975; Brunet, 1974).

Monamines (catecholamines, serotonin, melatonin) apparently affect prolactin secretion by altering the release of PIF or PRF from the hypothalamus (Meites, 1972, 1973; Tolis and Friesen, 1974). There seems also to be a direct effect of these agents on the pituitary (MacLeod and Lehmeyer, 1972; Meites, 1973).

As far as <u>target hormones</u> are concerned, it is well known that estrogen stimulates prolactin synthesis and releases both *in vivo* and *in vitro* (MacLeod and Lehmeyer, 1972; Meites, 1973; Tolis and Friesen, 1974) indicating that in addition to its well known action on the hypothalamus, estrogen has a <u>direct</u> action on pituitary cells. There is now both autoradiographic (Attramadal, 1970; Stumpf, Sar, and Keefer, 1975) and biochemical (Leavitt, Kimmel, and Friend, 1973) evidence that estrogen binds specifically to pituitary cells--especially nuclear components. Thus, its mechanism of action on pituitary cells is probably the same as that on peripheral target tissues (O'Malley and Means, 1974), and involves binding of the steroid to a specific cytoplasmic protein and migration of the steroid-binding-protein complex to the nucleus, where mRNA synthesis (transcription) is affected.

PROBLEMS REMAINING FOR THE FUTURE

The preceding outlines our present understanding of the cellular events involved in prolactin secretion and its control. A number of questions remain to be answered by future work; some of these are indicated below.

Is prolactin synthesized directly or is it synthesized as a precursor molecule which must be modified intracellularly prior to its discharge from the cell? We know that several polypeptide hormones, notably insulin and parathormone (see Tager and Steiner, 1974), are synthesized as larger, precursor molecules (proinsulin and proparathormone) which are cleaved proteolytically intracellularly prior to discharge from the cell. In the case of prolactin, different forms of the hormone have been detected by some (Swearingen, 1971; Nichols and Nicoll, 1974) but not by others (Zanini, Giannattasio, and Meldolsei, 1974; Kataoka, Imai, and Hollander, 1974). The cell fractionation studies of Zanini *et al.* (1974) suggest, but do not prove conclusively, that there are <u>no</u> precursor forms of the hormone. Therefore, this remains an unsettled issue.

Several other questions also remain to be satisfactorily answered: is exocytosis the only means of discharge of prolactin and other pituitary hormones? Are some hormone molecules (especially newly synthesized hormone molecules) preferentially released by a mechanism other than exocytosis? Work by Nicoll and Swearingen (1970), Swearingen (1971) and Labrie, Pelletier, Lemay, Borgeat, Barden, Dupont, Savary, Côté, and Boucher (1973) indicates that newly synthesized prolactin is preferentially released over old (stored) prolactin. These observations have sometimes been interpreted as indicating that some of the usual secretion steps, especially exocytosis of granules, may be by-passed. However, further studies are required to establish if this is the case or whether functional heterogeneity within the cell population could explain the findings.

Are microtubules and/or microfilaments involved in exocytosis? Further work is needed to establish such a connection because of the aforementioned multiple effects (especially on membranes) of the drugs used as probes of microtubule and microfilament function.

How is concentration accomplished? As already indicated, at present the nature of the processes by which prolactin is concentrated and insolubilized in secretory granules is not understood.

What triggers crinophagy? Nothing at all is known on this point just as nothing is known in general about what triggers fusions between other appropriate cellular organelles (e.g., phagosomes with lysosomes; peripheral Golgi vesicles with condensing vacuoles).

The answer to all these questions and many others are not presently available, but since the problems posed are currently under investigation in many laboratories they will undoubtedly be resolved in due time.

SUMMARY

The mammotroph or prolactin-secreting cell, due to its distinctive fine structure, large granules, and sustained survival *in vitro*, has been a favorite object for studying mechanisms of pituitary secretion and its control. In this review the structural basis of prolactin secretion is summarized and the proposed sequence of intracellular events involved in prolactin secretion together with their site of loaction is outlined. The available evidence validating the various steps in prolactin secretion and their regulation is summarized. Finally, some of the unresolved problems remaining for the future are pinpointed.

ACKNOWLEDGEMENT

The author wishes to express her thanks to Ms. Janet Pfeiffer and JoAnne Reid for their excellent technical assistance in this work, and to Ms. Lynne Wootton for her untiring secretarial assistance in the preparation of the manuscript.

Figures 1, 3, and 8-10 are reproduced with the permission of the Rickefeller University Press. Figures 5-7 are reproduced by the permission of the Cambridge University Press.

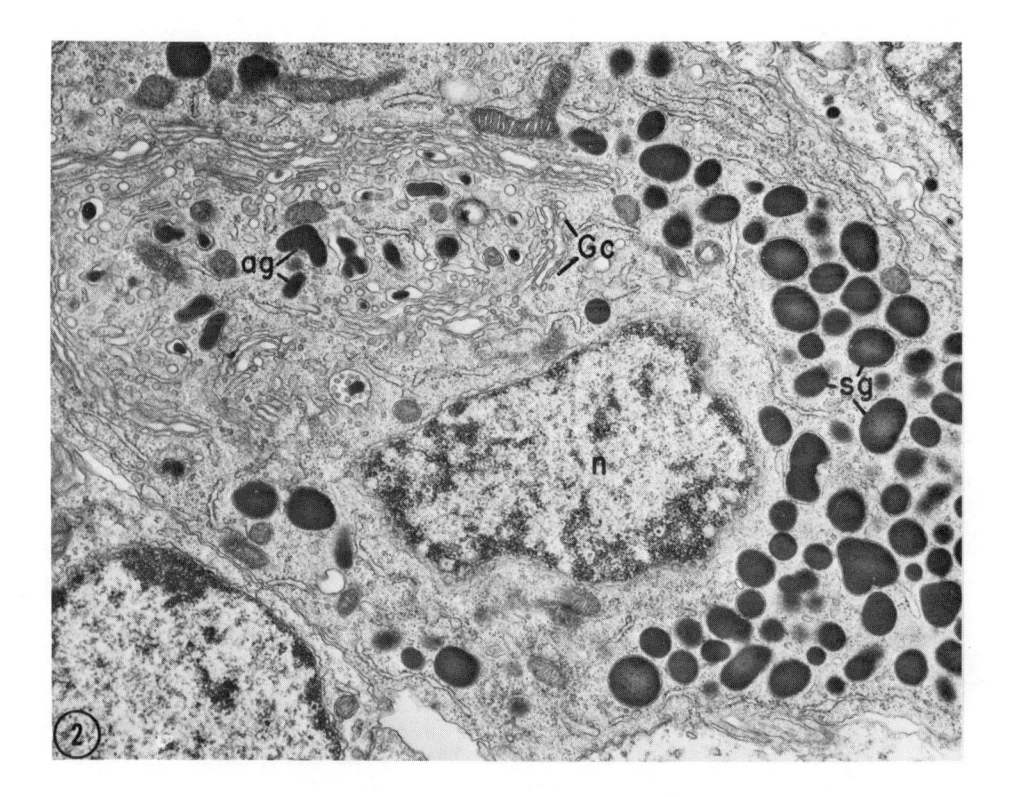

Figure 2. Mammotroph from a small block of pituitary tissue obtained from a male rat and incubated *in vitro* for 1 hr. The cell can be readily identified by its content of large, dense secretory granules which vary in size and shape. An accumulation of mature secretory granuels is seen to the right of the nucleus (n) at one pole of the cell, and the Golgi complex (Gc) which contains many immature granules is seen to the left at the opposite pole. The mature granules are larger (ranging from 500-800 nm maximal diameter) and are mostly round to ovoid in shape. The immature granules are smaller and polymorphous. X 13,000.

Figure 3. Mammotroph from the anterior pituitary gland of a lactating rat. This cell shows the typical morphological features associated with cells producing large quantities of proteins for export: abundant peripheral arrays of rough ER (er) parallel to the cell membrane (cm), a large population of attached polyribosomes and a large Golgi complex (Gc) containing many profiles of forming granules (ag). Immature granules vary in size and shape and are concentrated in the core of cytoplasm circumscribed by the Golgi cisternae. Mature granules are rounded or ovoid, more uniform in size (600-900 nm), and are found primarily between the Golgi complex and ER (at sg) or along the cell membrane (at sg^1). Numerous part rough- and part smooth transitional elements (te) of the ER are seen between the peripheral ER arrays and the Golgi complex. Clusters of smooth-surfaced vesicles (ve) are located in close proximity to the outer cisternae of the Golgi complex. These resemble in size and location similar vesicles found in the exocrine pancreatic cell and are thought to act as shuttle carriers to transport the secretory product from the rough ER to the Golgi elements. A single lysosome (ly) is present in the Golgi region. The inset depicts a polymorphous immature granule (ag) formed by the aggregation of several smaller granules. (See also Figs. 5 and 6). X 24,000; inset, X 40,000. (From Smith and Farquhar, 1966).

CELLULAR SECRETION AND CRINOPHAGY 59

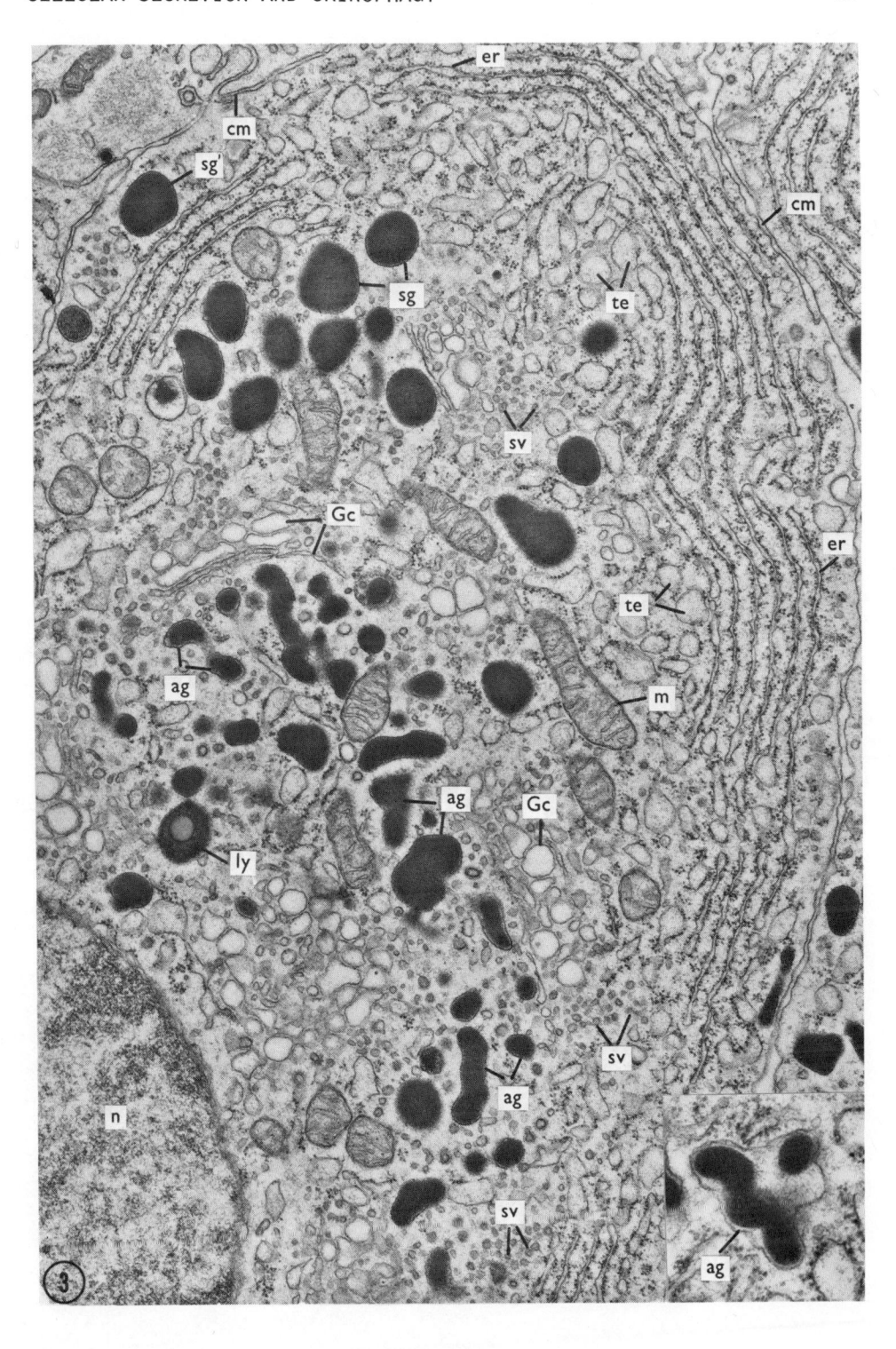

Figure 4. Parallel array of rough endoplasmic reticulum (er) in a mammotroph from a lactating animal. Abundant, closely-spaced, polyribosomes stud the outer surfaces of the membranes. In a number of places (arrows) the section cuts across the membranes in grazing section exposing the clusters of polyribosomes on their surface. ve, vesicles; sg, secretion granule. X 48,000.

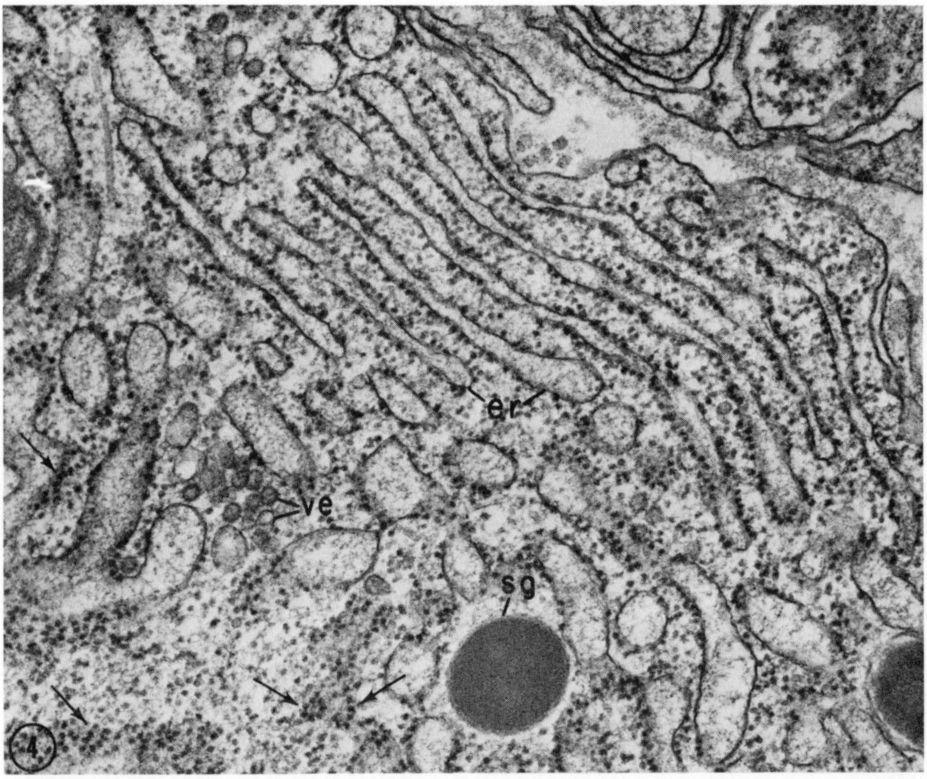
er
ve
sg
4

Figures 5 and 6. Portions of mammotrophs from lactating animals. In Fig. 5, a stack of three to five slightly curved Golgi cisternae (Gc) occupies the center of the field. The central core of cytoplasm circumscribed by the cisternae contains several immature secretion granules (ag). The outer cisternae along the convex surface of the Golgi stack are dilated or vacuolar whereas the inner ones (ic) along the concave surface of the Golgi stack are more flattened. Three small, rounded (100-200 nm) masses (arrows) of condensing secretory material are present within the innermost Golgi cisterna and another small granule (s) is seen along the concave Golgi surface. The polymorphous granules in the Golgi 'core' appear to be formed by fusion and aggregation of several of the smaller units which bud from the inner cisterna. Fig. 6 shows a group of these aggregating granules (ag_1-ag_3) in the Golgi region of another cell: ag_1 and ag_2 appear to have been formed by the fusion of three small granules, and ag_3 of multiple small granules. Note also that there is some dense material around the granule contents in ag_2 and ag_3. Mammotroph secretory granules appear to be formed in several steps: (a) small granules arise within the inner Golgi cisternae (arrows, Fig. 5); (b) these granules (s) pinch off and are found along the concave Golgi face; (c) several small granules merge to form larger aggregates (ag) of variable shape; and (d) these round up to form large (500-900 nm) ovoid or elliptical mature granules. m, mitochondria. Fig. 5, X 51,000; Fig. 6, X 63,000. (From Farquhar, 1971).

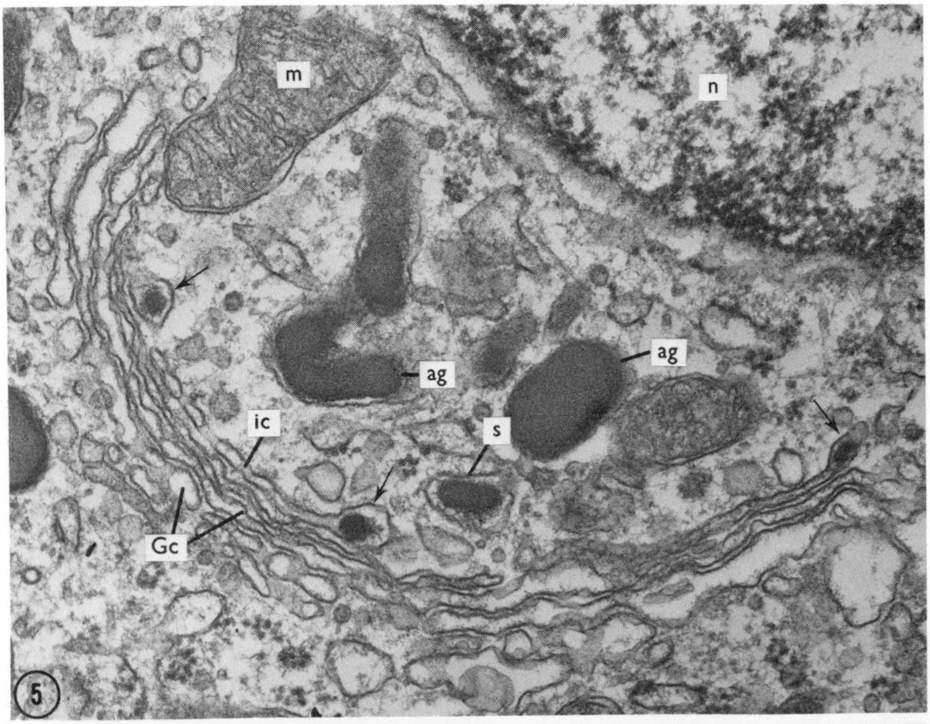
m
n
ag
ag
ic
s
Gc
5

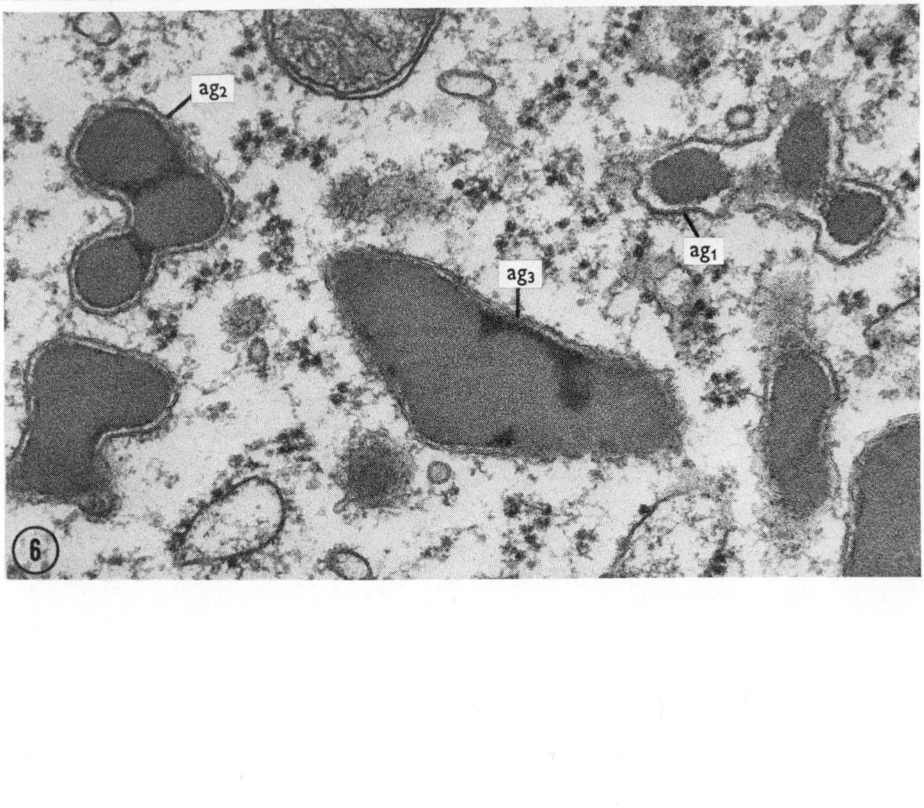
ag2
ag1
ag3
6

Figure 7. Peripheral cytoplasm of a mammotroph from a lactating rat, depicting several secretory granules (sg) lined up facing the perivascular spaces and undergoing discharge by exocytosis. The membranes of several granules are in continuity with the cell membrane at the points indicated by arrows. The content of the granules retains its characteristic shape and form momentarily after fusion. The one on the left, being smaller than the rest, may have already undergone partial solubilization. B, basement membrane; m, mitochondria. X 52,000. (From Farquhar, 1971).

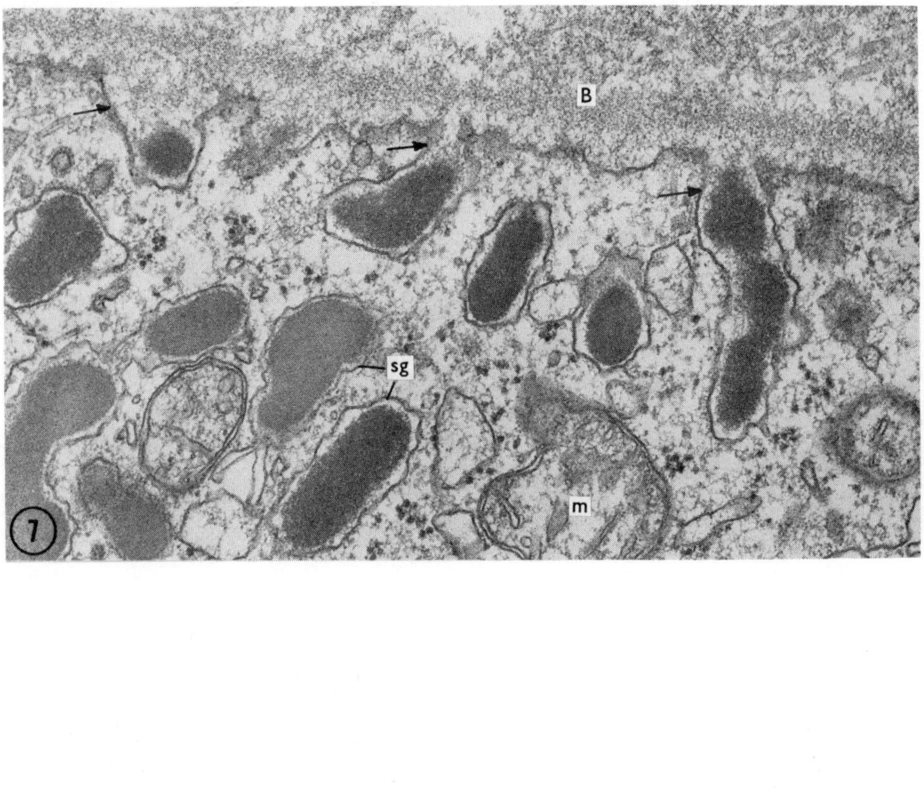
B
sg
m
7

Figures 8 - 10. Portions of mammotrophs of lactating rats sacrificed 24-48 hours after removal of suckling young, showing "crinophagy" or uptake of secretory granules into lysosomes. The field in Fig. 8 includes two lysosomes -- a multivesicular body (ly_1) and a dense body (ly_2). Both contain granules. The multilobulated mass in ly_1 appears to be derived rom an immature, aggregating granule. Fig. 9 shows another lysosome containing a large granule (gr). Fig. 10 is an acid phosphatase preparation, demonstrating the presence of lead phosphate reaction product for the enzyme as well as the content of a secretory granule in the same lysosome. Several secretory granules (sg) are also seen free in the cytoplasm. Note that whereas membranes are present around granules in the cytoplasm, none is present around the granule cores found in lysosomes. Upon fusion of the granule with the lysosome the granule membrane becomes incorporated into that of the lysosome. The granule contents do not immediately disperse but remain visible as discrete entities for an undefined period of time until they are presumably dispersed and digested by the lysosomal proteases present. m, mitochondria. Fig. 8, X56,000; Fig. 9, X 68,000; Fig. 10, X 75,000. (From Smith and Farquhar, 1966).

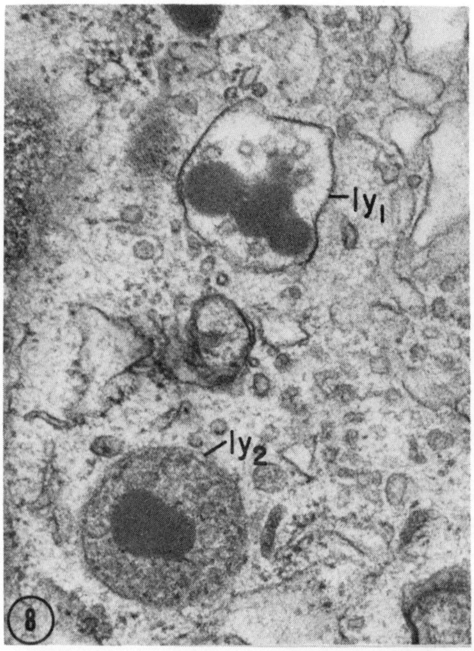

ly_1
ly_2
8

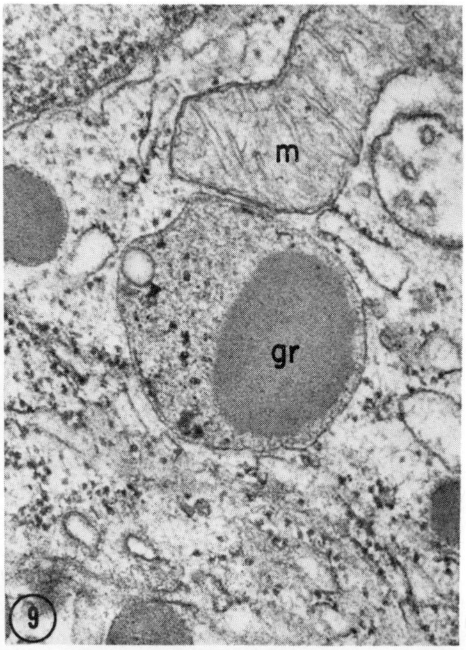

m
gr
9

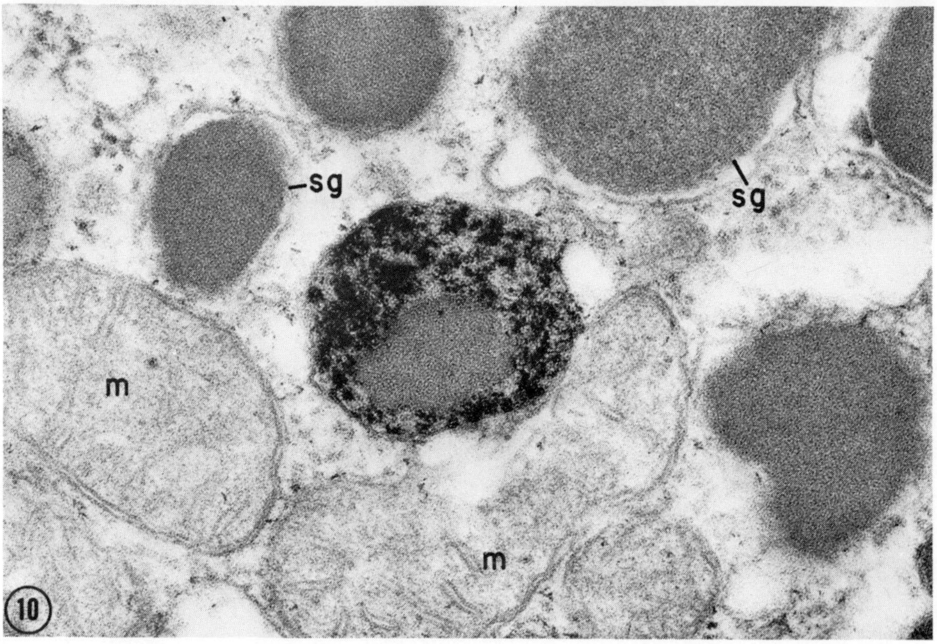

sg
sg
m
m
10

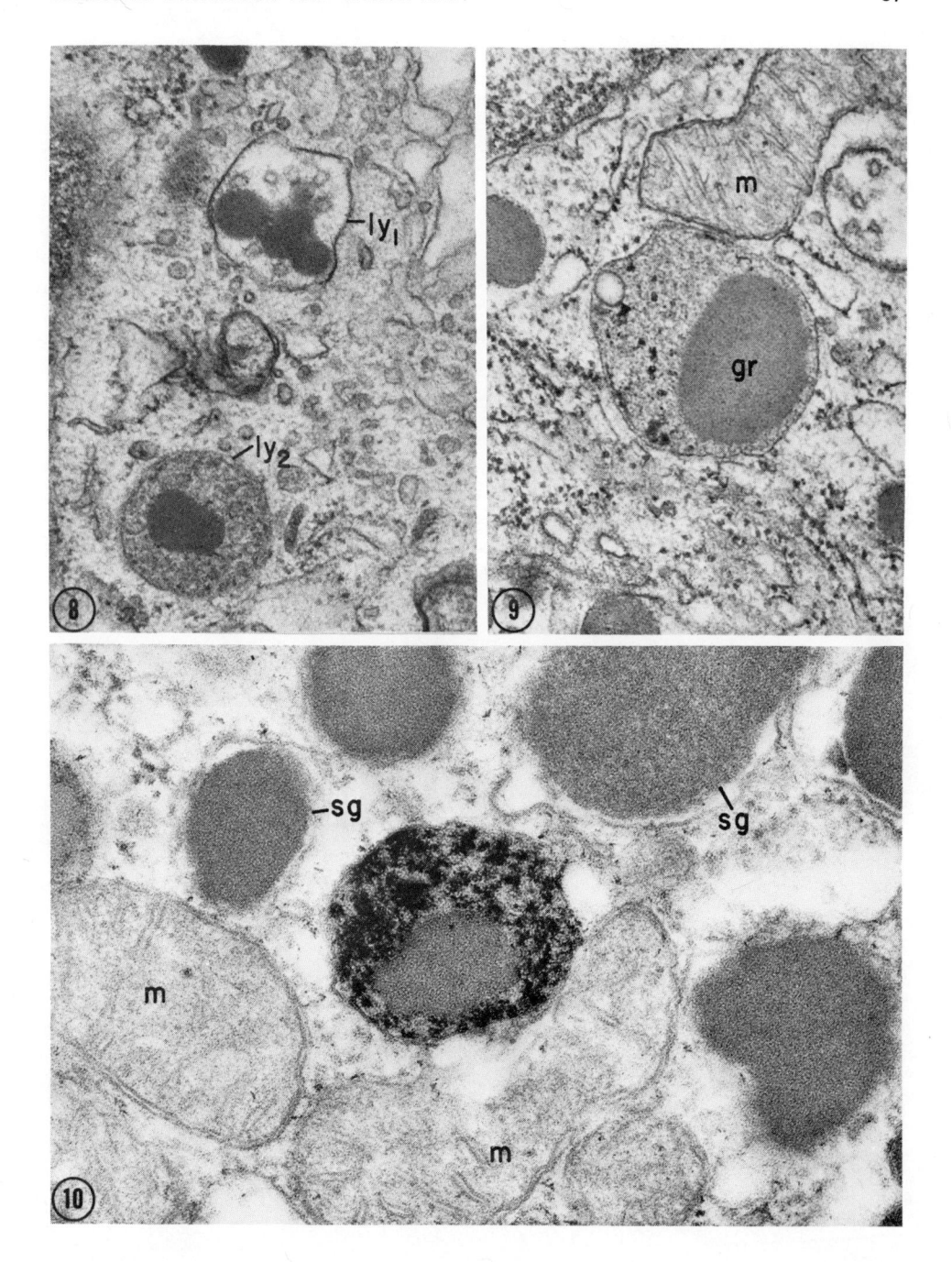

Figure 11. Mammotroph from a single cell suspension of pituitary cells. Suspensions were prepared by enzymatic dispersion (Hopkins and Farquhar, 1973) of pituitaries from estrogen-treated (5 µg/day for 5 days) female rats. The cell is rounded up and is easily identified by its content of large, secretory granules (sg). The nucleus (n) is located to one pole of the cell and the large Golgi complex (Go) is found on the other. The Golgi complex is highly developed and consists of 5-6 cisternae (c) with a content of low density which circumscribe a large circular area of the cytoplasm. X 13,000.

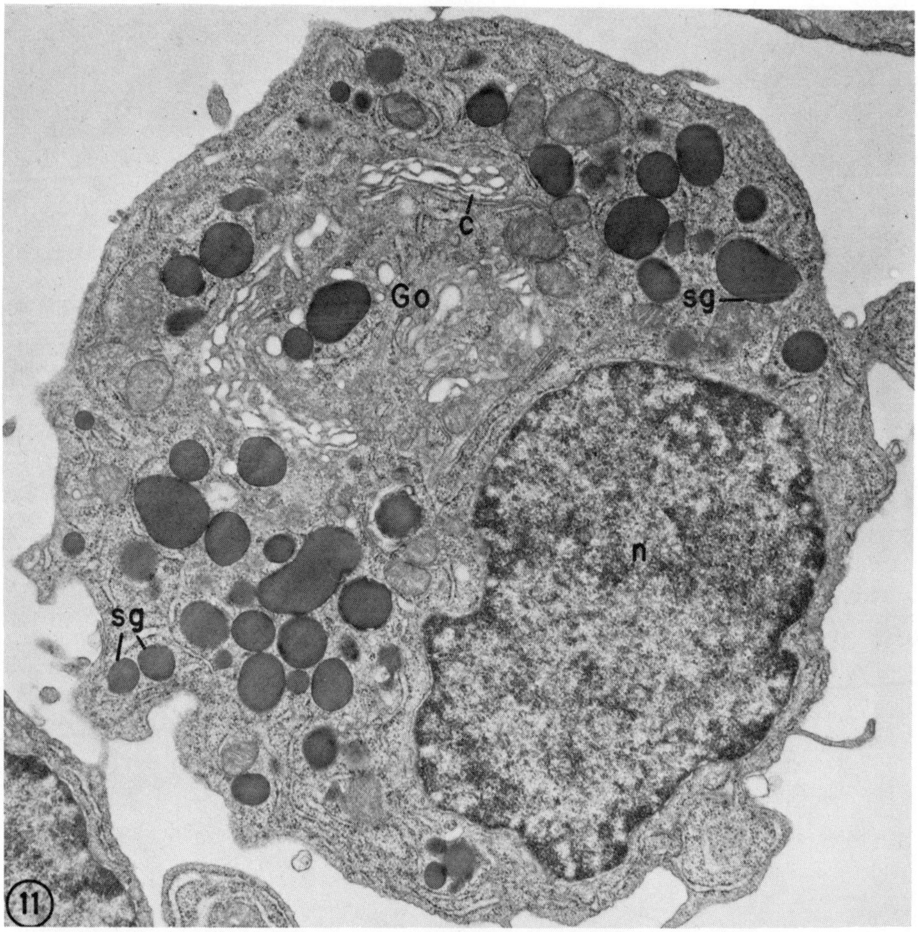
c
Go
sg
sg
n
11

Figure 12. Radioautogram of a mammotroph obtained from a pituitary of an estrogen-treated rat, cultured for 15 hours after dissociation and given a 5 min. leucine pulse, followed by a 1 min. chase incubation. The radioautographic grains are distributed over nucleus (n) and cytoplasm with the majority being associated with the rough ER (er). Go, Golgi region. X 14,000.

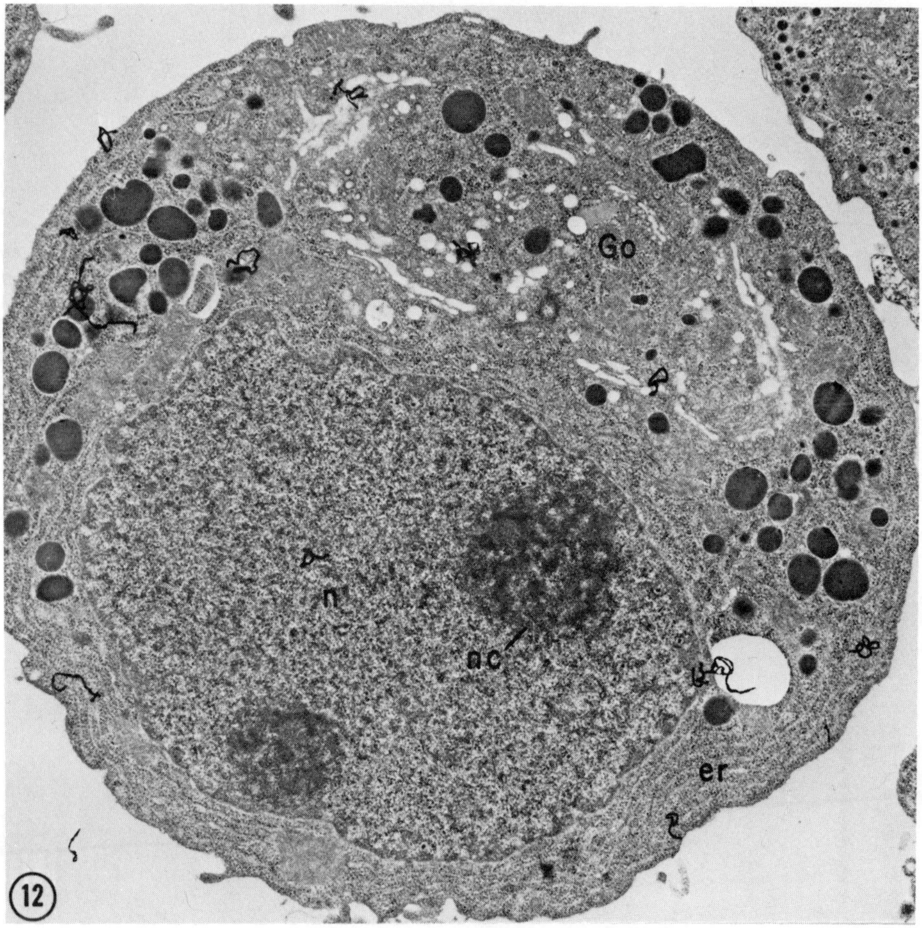
Go
n
nc
er
12

Figure 13. Radioautogram of a mammotroph prepared and pulsed as in Fig. 12, and fixed after a 20 min. chase incubation. Note that most of the grains are concentrated over the small (∼ 150 nm) forming granules along the inner (concave) surface of the Golgi complex (Gc) where it faces the nucleus (n). X 17,000.

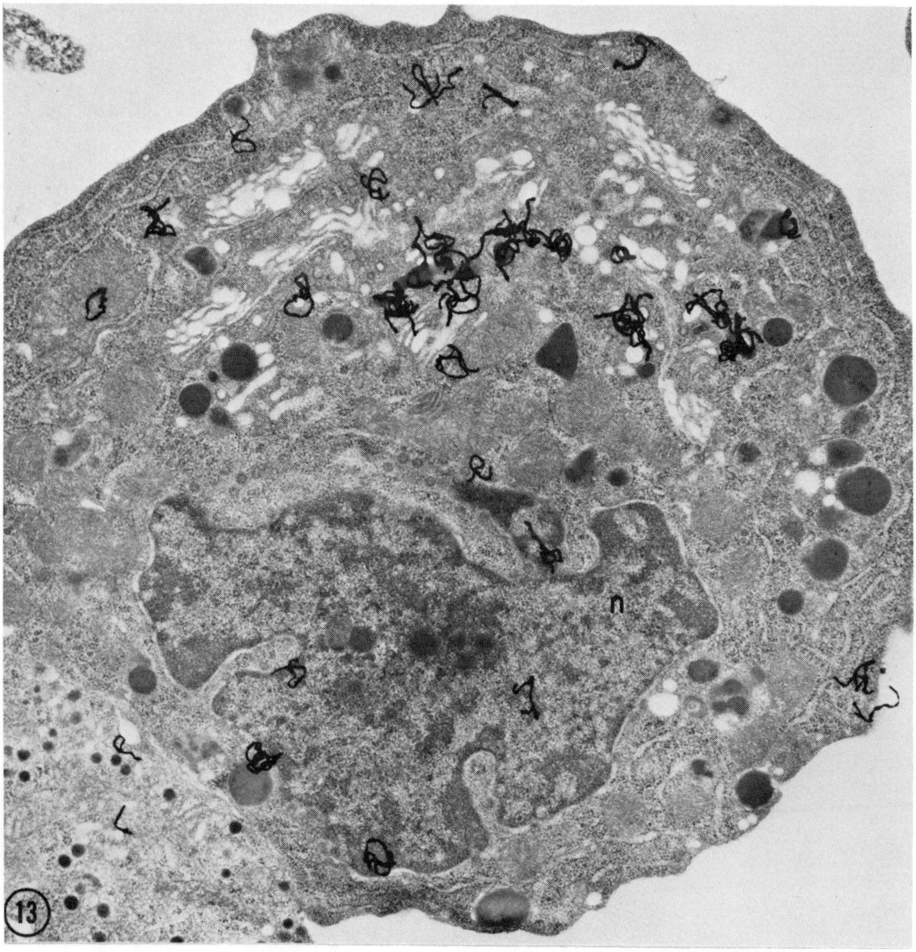
13
n

Figures 14 - 15. Preparations similar to that in Figs. 12-13, only fixed after a 1 hour chase incubation. Here the radioautographic grains are concentrated over the polymorphous, aggregating granules in the Golgi region (Go). Fig. 15 is an enlargement showing two such aggregating granules (ag) both of which show multiple radioautographic grains concentrated over them. Fig. 14, X 13,000; Fig. 15, X 30,000.

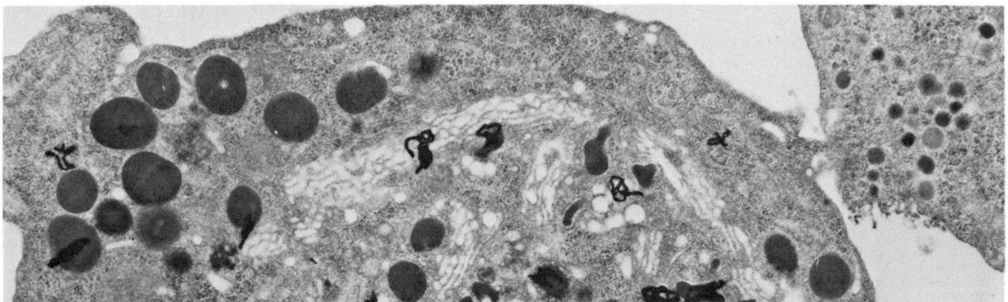
Go
14

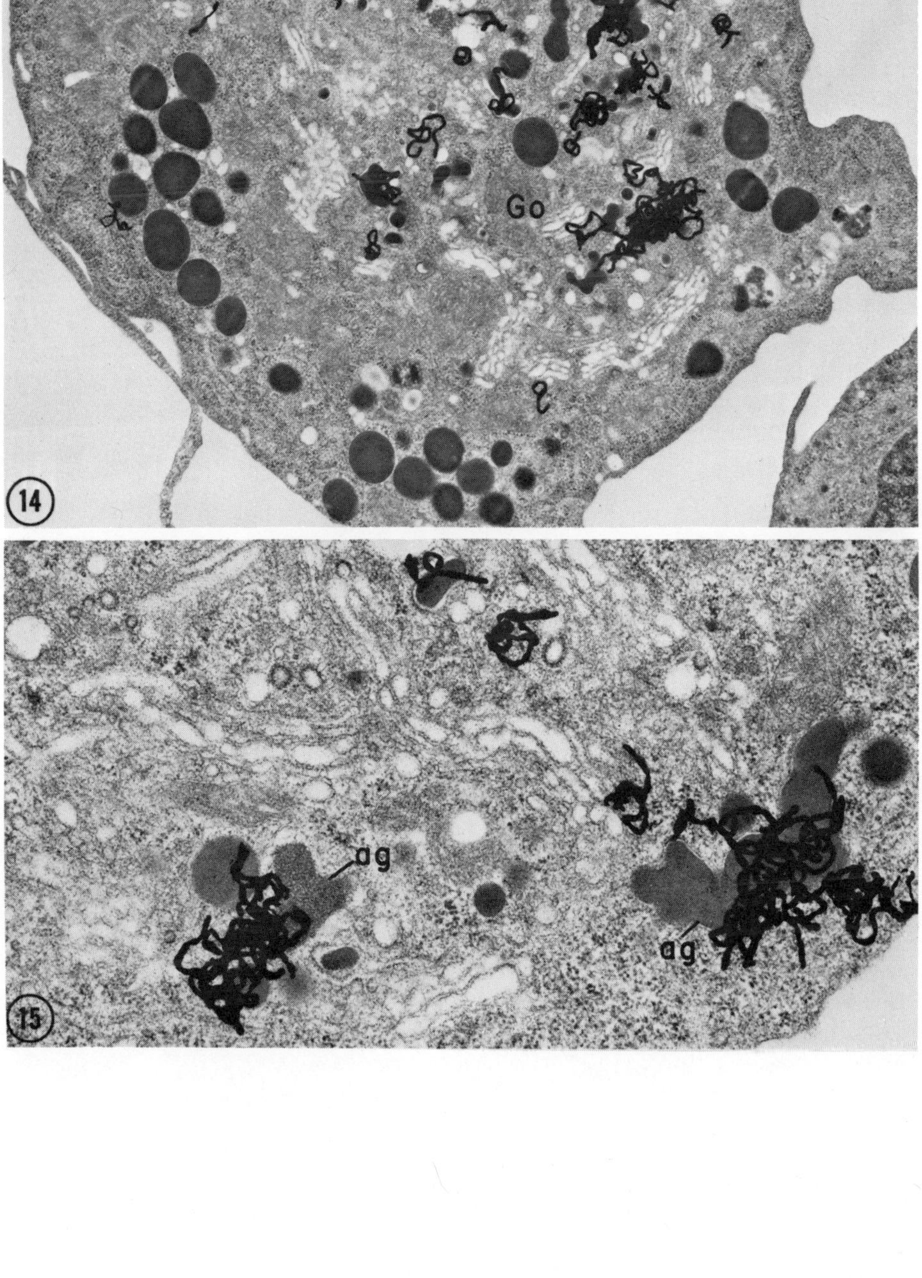
ag
ag
15

Figures 16 - 17. Radioautograms similar to those in the preceeding figures, only fixed after 2-3 hour chase incubation, showing concentrations of grains over mature secretion granules. In Fig. 16, taken after 2 hours, the grains are primarily over large granules which have an irregular shape, i.e., have not fully rounded up into the mature spherical or ovoid form. In Fig. 17, taken after 3 hours, the grains are concentrated over spherical, mature granules. Fig. 16, X 14,000; Fig. 17, X 17,000.

16

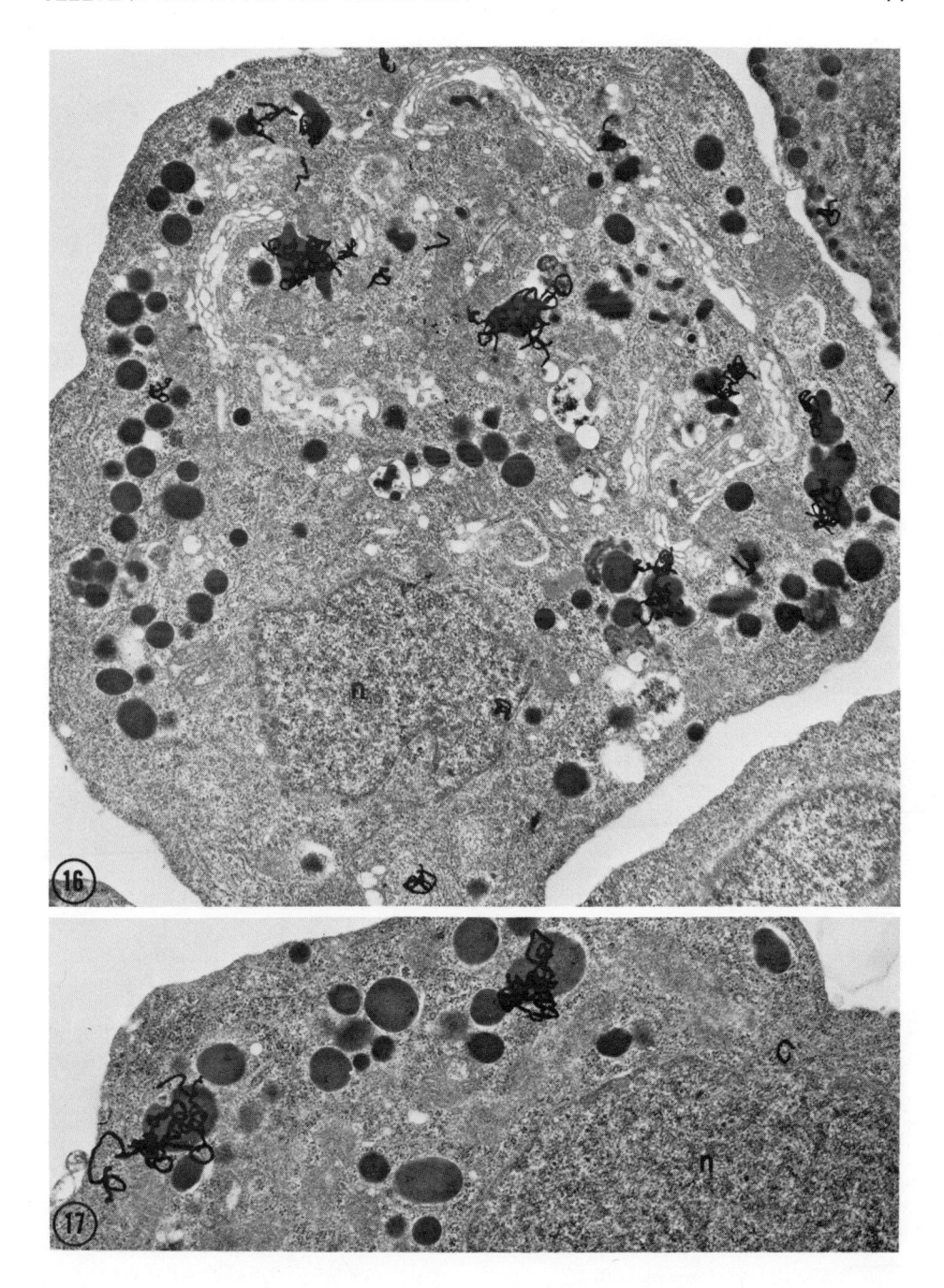

17

REFERENCES

Adiga, P.R., Hussa, R., Robertson, M., Hohl, H., and Winnick, T. (1968). Polysomes of bovine anterior pituitary gland and their role in hormone and protein biosynthesis. Proc. Natl. Acad. Sci., U.S.A. 60, 606-613.

Adiga, P.R., Hussa, R., and Winnick, T. (1968). Ribonucleoprotein particles of bovine anterior pituitary gland. Physiochemical and biosynthetic characteristics. Biochemistry 7, 1808-1817.

Adiga, P.R., Murthy, P., and McKenzie, J. (1971). Stimulation by adenosine 3',5'-cyclic monophosphate of protein synthesis by adenohypophysial polyribosomes. Biochemistry 10, 711-715.

Attramadal, A. (1970). Cellular localization of ^{3}H-oestradiol in the hypophysis. Z. Zellforsch. Mikrosk. Anat. 104, 597-614.

Baker, B.L. (1970). Studies on hormone localization with emphasis on the hypophysis. J. Histochem. Cytochem. 18, 1-8.

Baker, B.L., Midgley, A.R., Jr., Gersten, B.E., and Yu, Y. (1969). Differentiation of growth hormone and prolactin-containing acidophils with peroxidase-labeled antibody. Anat. Rec. 164, 163-171.

Biswas, D.K., and Tashjian, A.H. (1974). Intracellular site of prolactin synthesis in rat pituitary cells in culture. Biochem. Biophys. Res. Commun. 60, 241-248.

Bowers, C., Friesen, H.G., Hwang, P., Guyda, H.J., and Folkers, K. (1971). Prolactin and thyrotrophin release in man by synthetic pyroglutamyl-histidyl-prolinamide. Biochem. Biophys. Res. Commun. 45, 1033-1041.

Brunet, N., Gourdji, D., Tixier-Vidal, A., Pradelles, P., Morgat, J.L., and Fromageot, P. (1974). Chemical evidence for associated TRF with subcellular fractions after incubation of intact rat prolactin cells (GH$_3$) with ^{3}H-labeled TRF. FEBS Letters 38, 129-133.

Clementi, F., and Palade, G.E. (1969). Intestinal capillaries. I. Permeability to peroxidase and ferritin. J. Cell Biol. 56, 340-558.

Clementi, F., and Virgilis, G. (1967). Ultrastructure de l'adenohypophyse après ovariectomie et traitement par oestrogène et la progestérone. Path et Bact. 15, 119-131.

Costoff, A., and McShan, W.H. (1969). Isolation and biological properties of secretory granules from rat anterior pituitary glands. J. Cell Biol. 43, 564-574.

Couch, E.F., Arimura, A., Schally, A.V., Saito, M., and Sawano, S. (1969). Electron microscope studies of somatotrophs of rat pituitary after injection of purified growth hormone releasing factor (GRF). Endocrinology 85, 1084-1091.

Cuatrecasas, P. (1974). Membrane receptors. Ann. Rev. Biochem. 43, 169-214.

Dawson, A.B. (1946). Some evidences of specific secretory activity of the anterior pituitary gland of the cat. Am. J. Anat. 78, 347-410.

Dawson, A.B., and Friedgood, H.B. (1938). Differentiation of two classes of acidophils in the anterior pituitary gland of the female rabbit and cat. Stain Tech. 13, 17-21.

Ellis, S. (1960). Pituitary proteinase I: Purification and action on growth hormone and prolactin. J. Biol. Chem. 235, 1694-1699.

Farquhar, M.G. (1961a). Origin and fate of secretory granules in cells of the anterior pituitary gland. Trans N.Y. Acad. Sci. [2] 23, 346-351.

Farquhar, M.G. (1961b). Fine structure and function in capillaries of the anterior pituitary gland. Angiology 12, 270-292.

Farquhar, M.G. (1969). Lysosome function in regulating secretion: Disposal of secretory granules in cells of the anterior pituitary gland. In: *Lysosomes in Biology and Pathology*, Vol. 2, (Dingle, J.T. and Fell, H.B., eds.) pp. 462-482, North-Holland Publ., Amsterdam.

Farquhar, M.G. (1971). Processing of secretory products by cells of the anterior pituitary gland. Mem. Soc. Endocrinol. 19, 79-122.

Farquhar, M.G., and Rinehart, J.F. (1954). Electron microscopic studies of the anterior pituitary gland of castrate rats. Endocrinology 54, 516-541.

Farquhar, M.G., Skutelsky, E.H., and Hopkins, C.R. (1975). Structure and function of the anterior pituitary and dispersed pituitary cells. In vitro studies. In: The Anterior Pituitary, (Tixier-Vidal, A. and Farquhar, M.G., eds.) pp. 83-135, Academic Press, New York.

Gautvik, K.M., and Tashjian, A.H. (1973). Effects of cations and colchicine on the release of prolactin and growth hormone by functional pituitary tumor cells in culture. Endocrinology 93, 793-799.

Giannattasio, G., Zanini, A., and Meldolesi, J. (1975). Molecular organization of rat prolactin granules. I. In vitro stability of intact and "membraneless" granules. J. Cell Biol. 64, 246-250.

Gourdji, D., Tixier-Vidal, A., Morin, A., Pradelles, P., Morgat, J.L., Fromageot, P., and Kerdelhue, B. (1973). Binding of a tritiated thyrotropin releasing factor (TRF) to a prolactin secreting clonal cell line (GH3). Exp. Cell Res. 82, 39-46.

Grant, G., and Vale, W. (1974). Hypothalamic control of anterior pituitary hormone secretion -- characterized hypothalamic-hypophysiotropic peptides. In: *Current Topics in Experimental Endocrinology*, (James, V.H.T. and Martini, L., eds.) pp. 37-72, Academic Press, New York.

Grant, G., Vale, W., and Guillemin, R. (1972). Interaction of thyrotropin releasing factor with membrane receptors of pituitary cells. Biochem. Biophys. Res. Commun. 46, 28-34.

Guillemin, R., and Burgus, R. (1972). The hormones of the hypothalamus. Sci. Amer. 227 (Nov.), 24-33.

Hedinger, C.E., and Farquhar, M.G. (1957). Elektronenmikroskopische Untersuchungen von Zwei Typen acidophiler Hypophysenvorderlappenzellen bie der Ratte. Schweiz. Z. Pathol. Bakteriol. 20, 766-768.

Herlant, M. (1964). The cells of the adenohypophysis and their functional significance. Int. Rev. Cytol. 17, 299-382.

Hinkel, P.M., Woroch, E.L., and Tashjian, A., Jr. (1974). Receptor-binding affinities and biological activities of analogs of thyrotrophin-releasing hormone in prolactin-producing cells in culture. J. Biol. Chem. 249, 3080-3090.

Hopkins, C.R., and Farquhar, M.G. (1973). Hormone secretion by cells dissociated from rat anterior pituitaries. J. Cell Biol. 59, 276-303.

Hymer, W.C. (1975). Separation of organelles and cells from the mammalian adenohypophysis. In: *The Anterior Pituitary* (Tixier-Vidal, A. and Farquhar, M.G., eds.) pp. 137-180, Academic Press, New York.

Hymer, W.C., McShan, W.H., and Christiansen, R.B. (1961). Electron microscope studies of the anterior pituitary glands from lactating and estrogen-treated rats. Endocrinology 69, 81-90.

Hymer, W.C., Snyder, J., Wilfinger, W., Swanson, N., and Davis, J.A. (1974). Separation of pituitary mammotrophs from the female rat by velocity sedimentation at unit gravity. Endocrinology 95, 107-122.

Jacobs, L.S., Snyder, P.J., Wilber, J.F., Utiger, R.D., and Daughaday, W.H. (1971). Increased serum prolactin after administration of synthetic thyrotrophin releasing hormone (TRH) in man. J. Clin. Endocrinol. Metab. 33, 996-998.

Jamieson, J.D. (1972). Transport and discharge of exportable proteins in pancreatic exocrine cells: In vitro studies. Curr. Top. Membranes Transp. 3, 273-338.

Jamieson, J.D., and Palade, G.E. (1967a). Intrecellular transport of secretory proteins in the pancreatic exocrine cell. I. Role of the peripheral elements of the Golgi complex. J. Cell Biol. 34, 577-596.

Jamieson, J.D., and Palade, G.E. (1967b). Intracellular transport of secretory proteins in the pancreatic exocrine cell. II. Transport to condensing cavuoles and zymogen granules. J. Cell Biol. 34, 597-615.

Jamieson, J.D., and Palade, G.E. (1971a). Condensing vacuole conversion and zymogen granule discharge in pancreatic esocrine cells: metabolic studies. J. Cell Biol. 48, 503-522.

Jamieson, J.D., and Palade, G.E. (1971b). Synthesis, intracellular transport, and discharge of secretory proteins in stimulated pancreatic exocrine cells. J. Cell Biol. 50, 135-158.

Kataoka, K., Imai, Y., and Hollander, C.S. (1974). Absence of radioimmunoassayable precursors of prolactin in the pituitary of the rat. Abstracts, Fiftysixth Annual Meeting of the Endocrine Society, Atlanta, Georgia, A-183.

Kwa, A.A., Van der Gugten, A.A., and Ver hofstad, F. (1969). Radioimmunoassay of rat prolactin. Comparison of rat prolactin preparations isolated from the 'granular fraction' of pituitary tumor transplants and from normal pituitary glands. Brit. J. Cancer 5, 559-569.

LaBella, F., Krass, M., Fritz, W., Vivian, S., Shin, S., and Queen, G. (1971). Isolation of cytoplasmic granules containing growth hormone and prolactin from bovine pituitary. Endocrinology 89, 1094-1102.

Labrie, F., Barden, N., Poirier, G., and DeLean, A. (1972). Binding of thyrotropin releasing hormone to plasma membranes of bovine anterior pituitary gland. Proc. Nat. Acad. Sci. U.S.A. 69, 283-287.

Labrie, F., Beraud, G., Gauthier, M., and Lemay, A. (1971). Actinomycin-insensitive stimulation of protein synthesis in rat anterior pituitary *in vitro* by dibutyryl adenosine 3',5'-monophosphate. J. Biol. Chem. 246, 1902-1908.

Labrie, F., Gauthier, M., Pelletier, G., Borgeat, P., Lemay, A., and Gouge, J.J. (1973). Role of microtubules in basal and stimulated release of growth hormone and prolactin in rat adenohypophysis *in vitro*. Endocrinology 93, 903-914.

Labrie, F., Lamaire, S., and Courte, C. (1971). Adenosine 3',5'-monophosphate-dependent protein kinase from bovine anterior pituitary gland. I. Properites. J. Biol. Chem. 246, 7293-7302.

Labrie, F., Lemaire, S., Poirier, G., Pelletier, G., and Boucher, R. (1971). Adenohypophysial secretory granules. Their phosphorylation and association with protein kinase. J. Biol. Chem. 246, 7311-7317.

Labrie, F., Pelletier, G., Lemay, A., Borgeat, P., Barden, N., Dupont, A., Savary, M., Côté, J., and Boucher, R. (1973). 6th Symposium on Protein Synthesis in Reproductive Tissue. Karolinska Symposia on Research Methods in Reproductive Biology, 301-340.

Leavitt, W.W., Kimmel, G.L., and Friend, J.P. (1973). Steroid hormone uptake by anterior pituitary cell suspensions. Endocrinology 92, 94-103.

Lemaire, S., Pelletier, G., and Labrie, F. (1971). Adenosine 3',5'-monophosphate-dependent protein kinase from bovine anterior pituitary gland. II. Subcellular distribution. J. Biol. Chem. 246, 7303-7310.

Lemay, A., Deschenes, M., Lemaire, S., Poirier, G., Poulin, L., and Labrie, F. (1974). Phosphorylation of adenohypophyseal plasma membranes and properties of associated protein kinase. J. Biol. Chem. 249, 323-328.

Lemay, A., and Labrie, F. (1972). Calcium-dependent stimulation of prolactin release in rat pituitary *in vitro* by N^6-monobutyryl adenosine 3',5'-monophosphate. FEBS Letters 20, 7-10.

Lemay, A., Labrie, F., and Drouin, D. (1974). Stability of secretory granules containing growth hormone and prolactin from bovine anterior pituitary gland. Can. J. Biochem. 52, 327-335.

Li, C.H. (1972). Recent knowledge concerning the chemistry of lactogenic hormones. In: *Ciba Foundation Symposium on Lactogenic Hormones*, (Wolstenholme, G.E.W. and Knight, J., eds.) pp. 7-26, Churchill Livingstone, Edinburgh and London.

MacLeod, R.M., and Lehmeyer, J.E. (1972). Regulation of the synthesis and release of prolactin. In: *Ciba Foundation Symposium on Lactogenic Hormones*, (Wolstenholme, G.E.W. and Knight, J., eds.) pp. 53-82, Churchill Livingstone, Edinburgh and London.

MacLeod, R.M., Lehmeyer, J.E., and Bruni, C. (1973). Effect of antimitotic drugs on the *in vitro* secretory activity of mammotrophs and somatotrophs and on their microtubules. Proc. Sco. Exp. Biol. Med. 144, 259-267.

McDonald, J.K., Callahan, P.X., Ellis, S., and Smith, R.E (1971). Polypeptide degradation by dipeptidyl aminopeptidase I (cathepsin C) and related peptidases. In: *Tissue Proteinases*, (Barrett, A.J. and Dingle, J.T., eds.) pp. 69-107, North-Holland Publ., Amsterdam.

McShan, W.H., and Hartley, M.W. (1965). Production, storage and release of anterior pituitary hormones. Ergeb. Physiol., Biol. Chem. Exp. Pharmakol. 56, 264-296.

Meites, J. (1972). Hypothalamic control of prolactin secretion. In: *Ciba Foundation Symposium on Lactogenic Hormones*, (Wolstenholme, G.E.W. and Knight, J., eds.) pp. 325-338, Churchill Livingstone, Edinburgh and London.

Meites, J. (1973). Control of prolactin secretion in mammals. In: *International Symposium on Human Prolactin*, (Pasteels, R., ed.) pp. 105-118, American Elsevier Pub. Co., New York.

Meldolesi, J., Marini, D., and Marini, M.L.D. (1972). Studies on *in vitro* synthesis and secretion of growth hormone and prolactin. I. Hormone pulse labeling with radioactive leucine. Endocrinology 91, 802-808.

Moguilevsky, J.A., Cuerdo-Rocha, S., Christot, J., and Zambrano, D. (1973). The effect of thyrotrophic releasing factor on different hypothalamic areas and the anterior pituitary gland: A biochemical and ultrastructural study. J. Endocrinol. 56, 99-109.

Moriarty, G.C. (1973). Adenohypophysis: Ultrastructural cytochemistry. A review. J. Histochem. Cytochem. 21, 855-894.

Nagasawa, H., and Yanai, R. (1972). Promotion of prolactin release in rats by dibutyryl adenosine 3',5'-monophosphate. J. Endocrinol. 55, 215-216.

Nakane, P.K. (1970). Classifications of anterior pituitary cell types with immunoenzyme histochemistry. J. Histochem. Cytochem. 18, 9-20.

Nakane, P.K. (1975). Identification of anterior pituitary cells by immunocytochemistry. In: *The Anterior Pituitary*, (Tixier-Vidal, A. and Farquhar, M.G., eds.) pp. 45-61, Academic Press New York.

Nichols, C.W., Jr., and Nicoll, C.S. (1974). Secretion and metabolism of forms of rat adenohypophysial prolactin with different immuno- and bioactivities. Abstracts, Fifty-sixth Annual Meeting of the Endocrine Society, Atalnta, GA, A-184.

Nicoll, C.S., and Swearingen, K.C. (1970). Preliminary observations on prolactin and growth hormone turnover in rat adenohypophyses *in vitro*. In: *The Hypothalamus*. (Martini, L., Motta, M., and Fraschini, F., eds.) pp. 449-462, Academic Press, New York.

O'Malley, B.W., and Means, A.R. (1974). Female steroid hormones and target cell nuclei. Science 183, 610-620.

Palade, G.E. (1966). Structure and function at the cellular level. J. Amer. Med. Assn. 198, 815-825.

Palade, G.E. (1975). Intracellular aspects of the process of protein secretion. Science 189, 347-358.

Pantic, V., and Genbacev, O. (1972). Pituitaries of rats neonatally treated with estrogen. I. Luteotropic and somatotropic cells and hormones content. Z. Zellforsch. 126, 41-52.

Parsons, J.A. (1970). Effects of cations on prolactin and growth hormone secretion by rat adenohypophyses *in vitro*. J. Physiol. 210, 973-987.

Parsons, J.A., and Erlandsen, S.L. (1974). Ultrastructural immunocytochemical localization of protein in rat anterior pituitary by use of the unlabeled antibody enzyme method. J. Histochem. Cytochem. 22, 340-351.

Pasteels, J.L. (1963). Recherches morphologiques et experimentales sur la secretion de prolactin. Arch. Biol. 74, 439-553.

Pasteels, J.L. (1972). Morphology of prolactin secretion. In: *Ciba Foundation Symposium on Lactogenic Hormones* (Wolstenholme, G.E.W. and Knight, J., eds.) pp. 241-256, Churchill Livingstone, Edinburgh and London.

Pelletier, G., and Bornstein, M.B. (1972). Effect of colchicine on rat anterior pituitary gland in tissue culture. Exp. Cell Res. 70, 221-223.

Pelletier, G., Lemay, A., Béraud, G., and Labrie, F. (1972). Ultrastructural changes accompanying the stimulatory effect of N^6-monobutyryl adenosine 3',5'-monophosphate on the release of growth hormone (GH) prolactin (PRL) and adrenocorticotropic hormone (ACTH) in rat anterior pituitary gland *in vitro*. Endocrinology 91, 1355-1371.

Pelletier, G., Peillon, F., and Vila-Porcile, E. (1971). An ultrastructural study of sites of granule extrusion in the anterior pituitary of the rat. Z. Zellforsch. Mikrosk. Anat. 115, 501-507.

Pelletier, G., and Puviani, R. (1974). Permeability of capillaries to different tracers and uptake of horseradish peroxidase by the secretory cells in rat anterior pituitary gland. Z. Zellforsch. 147, 361-372.

Peterson, R.E., and Guillemin, R. (1974). The hormones of the hypothalamus. Am. J. Med. 57, 591-600.

Poirier, G., DeLean, A., Pelletier, G., Lemay, A., and Labrie, F. (1974). Purification of adenohypophyseal plasma membranes and properties of associated adenylate cyclase. J. Biol. Chem. 249, 316-322.

Purves, H.D. (1961). Morphology of the hypophysis related to its function. In: *Sex and Internal Secretions*, Vol. 1, (Young, W.C., ed.) pp. 161-238, Williams & Wilkins, Baltimore, MA.

Purves, H.D. (1966). Cytology of the adenohypophysis. In: *The Pituitary Gland*, Vol. 1, (Harris, G.W. and Donovan, B.T., eds.) p. 147, University of California Press, Berkeley.

Rao, P., Robertson, M., Winnick, M., and Winnick, T. (1967) Biosynthesis of prolactin and growth hormone in slices of bovine anterior pituitary tissue. Endocrinology 80, 1111-1119.

Redman, C.M., and Sabatini, D.D. (1966). Vectorial discharge of peptides released by puromycin from attached ribosomes. Proc. Nat. Acad. Sci. U.S.A. 56, 608-615.

Redman, C.M., Siekevitz, P., and Palade, G.E. (1966). Synthesis and transfer of amylase in pigeon pancreatic microsomes. J. Biol. Chem. 241, 1150-1158.

Sano, M. (1962). Further studies on the theta cell of the mouse pituitary as revealed by electron microscopy, with special reference to the mode of secretion. J. Cell Biol. 15, 85-97.

Schally, A.V., Arimura, A., and Kastin, A.J. (1973). Hypothalmic regulatory hormones. Science 179, 341-350.

Shiino, M., Arimura, A., Schally, A.V., and Rennels, E.G. (1972). Ultrastructural observations of granule extrusion from rat anterior pituitary cells after injection of LH-releasing hormone. Z. Zellforsch. Mikrosk. Anat. 128, 152-161.

Shiino, M., Williams, M.G., and Rennels, E.G. (1972). Ultrastructural observation of pituitary release of prolactin in the rat by suckling stimulus. Endocrinology 90, 176-187.

Shiino, M., Williams, M.G., and Rennels, E.G. (1973). Thyroidectomy cells and their response to thyrotrophin releasing hormone (TRH) in the rat. Z. Zellforsch. Mikrosk. Anat. 138, 327-332.

Smith, R.E., and Farquhar, M.G. (1966). Lysosome function in the regulation of the secretory process in cells of the anterior pituitary gland. J. Cell Biol. 31, 319-347.

Smith, R.E., and Farquhar, M.G. (1970). Modulation in nucleoside diphosphatase activity of mammotrophic cells of the rat adenohypophysis during secretion. J. Histochem. Cytochem. 18, 237-250.

Stadler, J., and Franke, W.W. (1974). Characterization of the colchicine binding of membrane fractions from rat and mouse liver. J. Cell Biol. 31, 319-347.

Stratmann, I.E., Ezrin, C., and Sellers, E.A. (1974). Estrogen-induced transformation of somatotrophs into mammotrophs in the rat. Cell Tiss. Res. 152, 229-238.

Stumpf, W.E., Sar, M., and Keefer, D.A. (1975). Localization of hormones in the pituitary: Receptor sites for hormones from hypophysial target glands and the brain. In: *The Anterior Pituitary* (Tixier-Vidal, A., and Farquhar, M.G., eds.) pp. 63-82, Academic Press, New York.

Swearingen, K.C. (1971). Heterogeneous turnover of adenohypophysial prolactin. Endocrinology 89, 1380-1388.

Tager, H.S., and Steiner, D.F. (1974). Peptide hormones. Ann. Rev. Biochem. 43, 509-538.

Tashjian, A.H., Jr., Bancroft, F.C., and Levine, L. (1970). Production of both prolactin and growth hormone by clonal strains of rat pituitary tumor cells. J. Cell Biol. 47, 61-70.

Tashjian, A.H., Jr., Barowsky, N.J., and Jensen, D.K. (1971). Thyrotrophin releasing hormone: Direct evidence for stimulation of prolactin secretion. Biochem. Biophys. Res. Commun. 43, 516-523.

Tashjian, A.H., Jr., and Hoyt, R.F., Jr. (1972). Transient controls of organ-specific functions in pituitary cells in culture. In: *Molecular Genetics and Developmental Biology* (Sussman, M., ed.) pp. 353-387, Prentice-Hall, New York.

Tesar, J.T., Koenig, H., and Hughes, C. (1969). Hormone storage granules in the beef anterior pituitary. J. Cell Biol. 40, 225-235.

Tixier-Vidal, A., and Picart, R. (1967). Etude quantitative par radioautographic au microscope électronique de l'utilization de la DL-leucine-^{3}H par les cellules de l'hypophyse du canard en culture organotypique. J. Cell Biol. 35, 501-519.

Tolis, G., and Friesen, H.G. (1974). The control of prolactin secretion. In: *Recent Studies of Hypothalamic Function* (Kederis, K., and Cooper, K.E., eds.) pp. 134-146, S. Karger, Basel.

Vale, W., Blackwell, R., Grant, G., and Guillemin, R. (1973). TFR and thyroid hormones on prolactin secretion by rat anterior pituitary cells in culture. Endocrinology 93, 26-33.

Vale, W., Grant, G., Amoss, M., Blackwell, R., and Guillemin, R. (1972). Culture of enzymatically dispersed anterior pituitary cells: Functional validation of a method. Endocrinology 91, 562-572.

Vila-Porcile, E., Olivier, L., and Racadot, O. (1973). Exocytose polarisée des corps residuels lysosomiaux des cellules à prolactin dans l'adénohypophyse de la Ratte en post-lactation. C.R. Acad. Sci. 276, 355-357.

Wilber, J.F., and Seibel, M.J. (1973). Thyrotropin-releasing hormone interactions with an anterior pituitary membrane receptor. Endocrinology 92, 888-893.

Wilson, L., Bamburg, J.R., Mizel, S.B., Grisham, L.M., and Creswell, K.M. (1973). Interaction of drugs with microtubule proteins. Fed. Proc. 33, 158-166.

Zambrano, D., and Deis, R.P. (1970). The adenohypophysis of female rats after hypothalamic oestradiol implants: an electron microscopic study. J. Endocrinol. 47, 101-110.

Zanini, A., and Giannattasio, G. (1974). Molecular organization of rat prolactin secretory granules. In: *Advances in Cytopharmacology*, Vol. 2, (Ceccarelli, B., Clementi, F., and Meldolesi, J., eds.) pp. 329-339, Raven Press, New York.

Zanini, A., Giannattasio, G., and Meldolesi, J. (1974). Studies on *in vitro* synthesis and secretion of growth hormone and prolactin. II. Evidence against the existence of precursor molecules. Endocrinology 94, 104-111.

DISCUSSION AFTER DR. FARQUHAR'S PAPER

Dr. Winnacker

Have there been any efforts to quantitate the contribution of crinophagy of prolactin in various conditions? Could prolactin inhibiting factors stimulate crinophagy?

Dr. Farquhar

Up to now no one has tried to obtain quantitative data on crinophagy. So far the only information we have is derived from morphologic observations which tell us that under conditions when secretion is suppressed (after removal of suckling young), crinophagy is a reasonably common event, whereas in normally lactating or cycling females it is much less frequent. Theoretically it should be possible to obtain quantitative data, but practically it would be difficult. Since we do not know how to trigger crinophagy *in vitro*, the experiments would have to be done *in vivo*, and I'm not sure how reliable the data would be.

As to your second question, it is certainly possible that prolactin inhibitory factors could stimulate crinophagy, but at the moment we have no information one way or another.

Dr. Jacobs

There are hypotheses about extragranular modes of release; if indeed such modes exist, almost by definition one would not be able to see them since they would occur by way of extragranular mechanisms. Recently Stachura and Frohman (1975) have presented some very interesting evidence, using a complicated double label system in *in vitro* rat pituitaries, that shows very early release of newly synthesized growth hormone; by the usual kind of biosynthetic and secretory timetable that we are used to thinking about, this probably occurs too early for the newly synthesized material to have been packaged. That's obviously only inferential. The question I have is: Have you had the opportunity to look at the morphologic appearance of isolated mammotrophs in response to a variety of secretagogues, some of which you have mentioned -- TRH in particular? I am also curious as to whether you have had the opportunity to look at mammotrophs after exposure to catecholamines *in vitro*?

Dr. Farquhar

Let me answer the last question first because it is the simplest. We have not so far looked at the effects of various stimulants on the porlactin cell. We intend to, but there have been other things to do in the meantime. As to the other question -- I'm of course familiar with the work of Stachura and Frohman (1972) on growth hormone biosynthesis and release. In their experiments they incubated pituitary pieces for three hours in ^{14}C-leucine followed by a one-hour incubation in ^{3}H-leucine. They showed that under certain conditions (in the presence of hypothalamic extracts) newly synthesized hormone (^{3}H-labeled) was preferentially released over old (^{14}C-labeled) stored hormone. However, we know from autoradiography that in both the prolactin cell (see text) and the growth hormone cell (Howell and Whitfield, 1973; Hopkins and Farquhar, 1973), by one hour the hormone has already been packaged into secretory granules. Therefore, what they are presumably looking at is preferential release of newly-made secretory <u>granules</u> (over old stored granules). Accordingly, it is not necessary to postulate that the usual packaging steps are bypassed. If we look at other systems, primarily exocrine systems, which have been probed in detail by combined morphologic, autoradiographic and cell fractionation studies, there is absolutely no known instance when a cell does not handle a secretory protein by synthesizing it and segregating it immediately, within minutes, into the rough ER. I believe the findings obtained so far in the prolactin cell and the growth hormone cell can be explained in terms of extablished mechanisms, and there is no need to propose the heretic idea, for which there is no evidence, of a secretory protein floating around free in the cell sol.

Dr. Jacobs

I didn't mean to imply that this was a major mechanism; I just think that the data that I have seen from his lab are convincing.

Dr. Farquhar

Right, but I gathered that you were suggesting that this data could imply that hormone was not discharged by exocytosis.

Dr. Jacobs

I think the implication is inherent in the data simply because of the time scale and the time interval.

Dr. Farquhar

As already indicated, I believe these authors are looking at preferential release of newly synthesized secretory granules and there is no eveidence that exocytosis is bypassed.

Dr. Jacobs

Yes. But he has no morphologic or autoradiographic observations. The only observation is that freshly synthesized hormone is identified by incorporation of radioactivity into immunoprecipitable hormone which finds its way into the extracellular medium at a very early point in time. I think that is an interesting possibility for the interpretation of this observation. It may be a very minor pathway if it exists, but it is the only evidence I know which is even halfway convincing that the possibility exists that such a mechanism may be operative.

Dr. Farquhar

Well, I still think until proven otherwise, we should assume that the discharge process operates by membrane fusion.

Dr. Barnawell

One could also propose that crinophagy might be the mechanism whereby the cell fragments the prohormone, or treats the prohormone, and that this might be a possible route. I realize that you have at least in part answered that with the Italian workers proposal, but I assume this is the only evidence we have so far. Is it possible to go around the other way?

Dr. Farquhar

We answered it to our satisfaction initially, when we did this work, by the timescale of the observations. That is, if you look at animals with normally suckling young, you find primarily images of exocytosis. If you do Pasteel's experiment and take away the mothers and then put them back with the young, massive exocytosis of granules into the capillaries is found. If you take away the babies for 24-48 hours you see many images of crinophagy. Hence, the crinophagy process is visualized primarily under those circumstances when you shut off secretion by taking away the suckling young. So the physiology, plus the morphologic observations made us conclude that crinophagy is the mechanism for taking care of overproduction of secretory products rather than a mechanism for their activation. This association held up for all the other

CELLULAR SECRETION AND CRINOPHAGY

pituitary cell types. When you stimulate them you see primarily exocytosis, when you suppress them you see increased crinophagy.

Dr. Meites

Dr. Farquhar, I am puzzled by the slide showing the synthesis and release of the hormone. There are still at least two barriers for the granule, I noticed, both the cell surface and the capillary barrier, the membrane. You didn't tell us how the granule managed to get through these two barriers. Related to that, I wonder if you've done any work with any of the ergot drugs which have been shown to cause accumulation of granules at the inner membrane surface of the cell and whether you can tell us how the door is shut, so to speak, to prevent these granules from getting out.

Dr. Farquhar

We just don't have any answers to the last question, since we have not worked with ergot drugs. I suspect that if one looked all you would see is granule accumulation, and that wouldn't be too helpful in providing answers to mechanisms. As far as discharge of granules is concerned, I am glad you gave me the chance to point out what is known here. In the exocytosis slide I showed, you could see the granule content, at the time when the granules have just fused and you still have invaginating pockets with just their mouths open. Shortly after fusion they disappear from view; the hormone is apparently rapidly solubilized. Then presumably the solubilized hormone is able to simply diffuse through the remaining barriers to reach the capillary lumen. In order to get to the capillary lumen the hormone has simply to penetrate two basement membranes, one on the epithelial side and one on the capillary side, the connective tissue space between, and pass through the fenestrae of the endothelium. Endothelia of the pituitary and other endocrine glands are all provided with fenestrae which are about 500 Angströms in width and are covered by thin diaphragms. These diaphragms do not represent extensions of the cell membrane but as far as we know are composed of some glycoprotein or polysaccharide material strung across this gap. We know from the work of Clementi and Palade that a tracer such as horseradish peroxidase, which is about 40,000 in molecular weight, has no trouble penetrating from the capillary lumen, through these fenestrae, across the connective tissue layers to arrive at the cell membrane. So if substances of this molecular weight have no trouble, then we presume that pituitary hormones, which are something less than 30,000 MW, have no difficulty passing through these same barriers in the reverse direction. The main purpose for exocytosis is that you have to have a mechanism for transporting the hormone across the cell membrane in order to release it into perivascular space. Since we know that the cell membrane is impermeable to milecules over 200 MW, polypeptides have to be taken or ferried across in vesicles or in membrane-limited compartments by membrane fusion and fission. That is why it is implausible to think of hormones floating around freely in the cell

sol since they would be unable to cross the cell membrane and be
discharged.

Dr. Jacobs

Dr. Farquhar, I wonder if you would be willing to share with
us your thoughts or speculations about the mechanisms of dissolution
of this compacted hormone as it reaches the cell membrane. There
is fusion of the granule membrane with the cell membrane; we see
electron-dense stainable material, at least some, and perhaps most
of which, is hormone contained within these granules. Yet, as you
have shown, and as has been shown in other secretory tissues, it
is very rarely that one sees any dense material beyond the cell
membrane. Occasionally in the islet beta cell one might see what
looks like dissolving material, and I have certainly seen it in the
pituitary also occasionally, but it is not very common. Presumably,
as you have said, the contents of the granules simply dissolve, very
promptly, upon hitting the perivascular space. In the past you and
Dr. Smith have shown histochemically certain enzymes on a variety
of membranes, including granule membranes, if I remember correctly.
I wonder if there isn't some kind of an enzymatic activation process
important for granule dissolution, which takes place coincidentally
with the fusion of membranes. The reason I wonder about that is,
if one does a cell fractionation experiment and puts isolated
granules in a buffer designed to simulate extracellular fluid, they
sit there and stare at you; they don't dissolve in the least, at
least in my hands. One begins to wonder if the granules aren't a
bit like time bombs; they may have built-in mechanisms for their
own dissolution. Do you have any thoughts or speculations along
these lines?

Dr. Farquhar

Well, it would have to be just that - thoughts and speculations
- because we don't have any information. In the case of prolactin
granules, what we can say is that this material in the granule is
peculiarly stable, compared to other pituitary hormone granules.
It requires urea treatment or treatment in SDS in order to solubilize
the granule contents, as has been shown by the studies of Giannattasio and co-workers (1975). Recently these same workers have
succeeded in stripping off the membrane with mild detergents,
leaving the intact cores. If we knew how the cell succeeded in
making the concentrated, stable package, maybe we would know more
how it succeeds in disrupting it later. But certainly the mechanisms
that come to mind are the ones which you already described, that is,
the possibility that there is an enzyme or enzymes packaged with
the granule that trigger fusion and/or solubilization. It is also
possible that in the environment of the perivascular space there
are the appropriate agents which would promote solubilization. You
have just pinpointed some more interesting problems for the future
indicating that we still have some work to do.

CELLULAR SECRETION AND CRINOPHAGY

Dr. Dellmann

We have noticed that when we stimulate hypothalamic neurosecretory cells we get, together with an increased synthetic activity and production of neurosecretory granules which are transported down into the hypophysis, an increased crinophagy. I am wondering whether you have observed similar events in the prolactin cells. You mentioned that as soon as you shut off the stimulus you get crinophagy, but do you get it even before you shut off the stimulus?

Dr. Farquhar

In mammotrophs and other pituitary cells, you always see a low level of crinophagy going on, which to me isn't surprising. I suppose the cell is continually overproducing, so you can find images or crinophagy in normally secreting cells. In the lactating animals which are under this extreme discharge pressure such images are not very frequent. I think that one interesting point which was brought up is that in some other systems, lysosomes may participate in the activation of hormones. The most notable system where this has been shown is in the thyroid gland where the cell makes a large protein (thyroglobulin), which is subsequently degraded in lysosomes to produce active hormones (T_3 and T_4) - as follows: Thyroglobulin is synthesized, stored in the follicular lumen as colloid, and when hormone is needed, the colloid is reabsorbed as a droplet, the droplet fuses with a lysosome, the thyroglobulin is split by lysosomal proteases, and T_4 and T_3 are released. So here is a clear example of where lysosomes are used to produce the active form of the hormone. There may be other such instances. We don't have the full story yet on exactly where in the cell the prohormones, proparathormone and proinsulin, are activated. However, there is no reason to assume that this particular mechanism is exactly the same in all cell types. The prolactin cell is different from the thyroid cell, which may be different from the pancreatic beta cell, and in your situation it may be still different.

Dr. Dellmann

I think we may have a similar system in the neurosecretory cell because we see many lysosomes in the distal protion where discharge occurs, so that lysosomes may very well have some function in the secretory process. My next question is: Do you know what happens to the granular membrane when exocytosis occurs?

Dr. Farquhar

That is a popular question. Many people are trying to answer that, and perhaps I can just mention what we know so far. Once again, the problem has been looked at in the pituitary as well as in other systems. Dr. Pelletier and our group have looked at it in pituitary cells by trying to label the ourside membrane with a tracer such as horseradish peroxidase and then following what would happen to the membrane upon stimulation of discharge. It is clear that if all the granules are discharged into the cell surface and nothing is done about their membranes, the cell size would increase, and the pituitary would enlarge in size. Since the cell and gland size remain constant, we know we have to get rid somehow of the excess membrane of the released granules, and we looked for ways in which this might be done. Both Dr. Pelletier (1973) and our group (Farquhar, 1975) found evidence that at least a part of this material was being recovered intact (in the form of small vesicles) and recirculated back to the Golgi apparatus. In our studies on somatotrophs we found it in particular back in the inner Golgi cisterna, which is the site where the granules originally came from. There is also evidence from the work of Amsterdam et al. (1969) indicating part of the membrane is recovered intact. If the parotid is very intensely stimulated with isoproterenol, the secretory granules are completely depleted and in the process, a huge amount of membrane is relocated to the cell surface. There follows a recovery period when the cell membrane gradually decreases in size, and during this period a profusion of small vesicles is found in the cell, which appear to represent the mechanism for recovering membrane from the cell surface. So there is evidence that some of the membrane is recovered intact. At the moment we don't know whether or not some of it is also broken down. To summarize, we can say that the cell takes care of the situation by removing part of the membrane intact, but at the moment, we don't know just how much is removed in this manner and what other mechanisms may exist for its removal.

Dr. Parsons

We have wondered why we can't see prolactin in sites other than in the storage granules of prolactin cells by using ultra-structural immunocytochemical techniques (Parsons and Erlandsen, 1974), and we thought that we were losing the prolactin during fexation and dehydration. We have tried freeze-dried preparations where the tissues never came into contact with solvents other than the plastic embedment medium. When these freeze-dried tissues were evaluated along with traditionally fixed material, reaction products were localized only over secretion granules in both cases. These results may reflect problems associated with our techniques, however, we have been unsuccessful in our attempts to localize prolactin in the cisternae of the ER, the perivascular spaces, or anywhere other than in secretion granules.

Dr. Farquhar

I would like to know whether you know what the mechanism is of immunogenicity. In other words, what organization of the molecule determines the immunogenicity? The reason I asked that question is that we know now from work on a variety of cells that while the initial biosynthesis of proteins occurs at the level of the ribosome -- probably at the moment when the protein is synthesized -- other secondary modifications occur within the Golgi complex. There, for example, the terminal sugars and sulfur are added and certain molecular rearrangements take place. So the possibility exists that there is some addition or molecular arrangement occurring during passage through the Golgi apparatus that could explain the immunogenicity at this level and the lack of it in the ER.

Dr. Parsons

We were aware of that possibility and we suggested it in our recent manuscript (Parsons and Erlandsen, 1974). Studies on the beta cell in the pancreas may provide insight into the problems associated with the ultrastructural localization of hormones. Recently, Smith and van Frank (1974) showed by ultrastructural cytochemical techniques that the enzyme necessary for cleaving insulin from the proinsulin molecule is located in the secretion granules. Most interestingly, we have been unable to visualize insulin in sites other than the secretion granules in our immunocytochemical evaluation of beta cells as well (Erlandsen et al., 1974). Perhaps the appropriate immunogenicity is conferred after it has been cleaved from the proinsulin molecule.

Dr. Farquhar

Yes, I believe Bob Smith's work suggests that activation of the prohormone to hormone occurs primarily in immature granules, since that is where he found the enzyme to be located. If so, that would be another variation of the general secretion theme that I think is very interesting. It shows how innovative cells are.

DISCUSSION REFERENCES

Amsterdam, A., Ohad, I., and Schramm, M. (1969). Dynamic changes in the ultrastructure of the acinar cell of the rat parotid gland during the secretory cycle. J. Cell Biol. 41, 753-773.

Clementi, F., and Palade, G.E. (1969). Intestinal capillaries. I. Permeability to peroxidase and ferritin. J. Cell Biol. 41, 33-58.

Erlandsen, S.L., Parsons, J.A., Burke, J.P. and Van Orden, L.S. (1974). Immunocytochemical localization of insulin and glucagon on ultrathin sections for electron microscopy using the unlabeled antibody enzyme method. Program of the Thirty-fourth Annual Meeting of the American Diabetes Association, p. 339 (Abs. #9).

Farquhar, M.G., and Cheng, H. (1975). The presence of adenylate cyclase in Golgi fractions from rat liver (abstract). Anatomical Record 181, 330-331.

Giannattasio, G., Zanini, A., and Meldolesi, J. (1975). Molecular organization of rat prolactin granules. I. *In vitro* stabilization of intact and "membraneless" granules. J. Cell Biol. 64, 246-250.

Hopkins, C.R., and Farquhar, M.G. (1973). Hormone secretion by cells dissociated from rat anterior pituitaries. J. Cell Biol. 59, 277-303.

Howell, S.L., and Whitfield, M. (1973). Synthesis and secretion of growth hormone in the rat anterior pituitary. I. The intracellular pathway, its time course and energy requirements. J. Cell Sci. 12, 1-21.

Parsons, J.A., and Erlandsen, S.L. (1974). Ultrastructural immunocytochemical localization of prolactin in rat anterior pituitary by use of the unlabeled antibody enzyme method. J. Histochem. Cytochem. 22, 340-351.

Pelletier, G. (1973). Secretion and uptake of peroxidase by rat adenohypophyseal cells. J. Ultrastruct. Res. 43, 445-459.

Smith, R.E., and Van Frank, R.M. (1974). Substructural localization of an enzyme in β cells of rat pancreas with the ability to convert proinsulin to insulin. Proceedings of the Fifth-sixth Annual Meeting of the Endocrine Society, p. A-190 (Abs. #269).

Stachura, M.E., Dhariwal, A.P.S., and Frohman, L.A. (1972). Growth hormone synthesis and release in vitro: effects of partially purified ovine hypothalamic extract. Endocrinology 91, 1071-1078.

Stachura, M.E., and Frohman, L.A. (1975). Growth hormone: Independent release of big and small forms from rat pituitary in vitro. Science 187, 447-449.

THE ASSAY AND REGULATION OF PROLACTIN IN HUMANS

Andrew G. Frantz

Department of Medicine
College of Physicians and Surgeons of Columbia University
New York, New York 10032

The early advances in animal prolactin physiology outlined by Dr. Turner were not paralleled at that time by any corresponding advances in the study of human prolactin. The reasons for this were twofold: first, there was no clear indication until a few years ago that human beings possessed a prolactin which was definitely distinct from growth hormone. Human growth hormone and primate growth hormone have intrinsic prolactin activity, unlike non-primate growth hormones, and early efforts to isolate a separate human prolactin were unsuccessful. The second problem was that the existing prolactin bioassays at that time were too insensitive to be applied successfully to the study of prolactin in human blood.

The following review will focus on recent developments in the assay of human prolactin and what has been learned from it regarding the regulation of the hormone in man. The major emphasis will be on work from the author's laboratory and animal studies will not be mentioned except in passing.

ASSAY

Bioassay

The first attempts to examine the question of human prolactin in this laboratory were aimed at developing an assay more sensitive than that of the standard pigeon crop sac (Riddle, Bates, and Dykshorn, 1933). The preparation which we began to examine was that of the mouse breast in organ culture. This was a system which had been explored for many years by a number of investigators (Hardy, 1950; Elias, 1957; Rivera and Bern, 1961; Juergens, Stockdale, Topper and

Elias, 1965; Topper, 1968), and its hormonal requirements for differentiation and for milk production *in vitro* had been well established, but it had not previously been used for assay purposes or applied to the study of human blood. Almost as soon as we began to look at this system it became evident that it was responsive to prolactin at doses considerably below what earlier studies would have suggested (Frantz and Kleinberg, 1970; Kleinberg and Frantz, 1971).

Figure 1 shows the appearance of mouse breast tissue from a 9-day pregnant animal, incubated in medium 199 to which had been added insulin, 10 µg/ml, hydrocortisone, 20 µg/ml, and also 30% pooled male plasma. An early finding was that not only is the system tolerant of plasma in the medium, but the presence of plasma seems to stabilize it, reducing the incidence of necrosis, and considerably enhances the responsiveness to small amounts of added ovine prolactin. Figure 2 shows the same tissue from the same animal with ovine prolactin at a dose of 50 ng/ml in the medium. There is a very pronounced secretory response with essentially all of the lumina being distended with dark red staining secretory material, representing the various milk proteins. These responses are

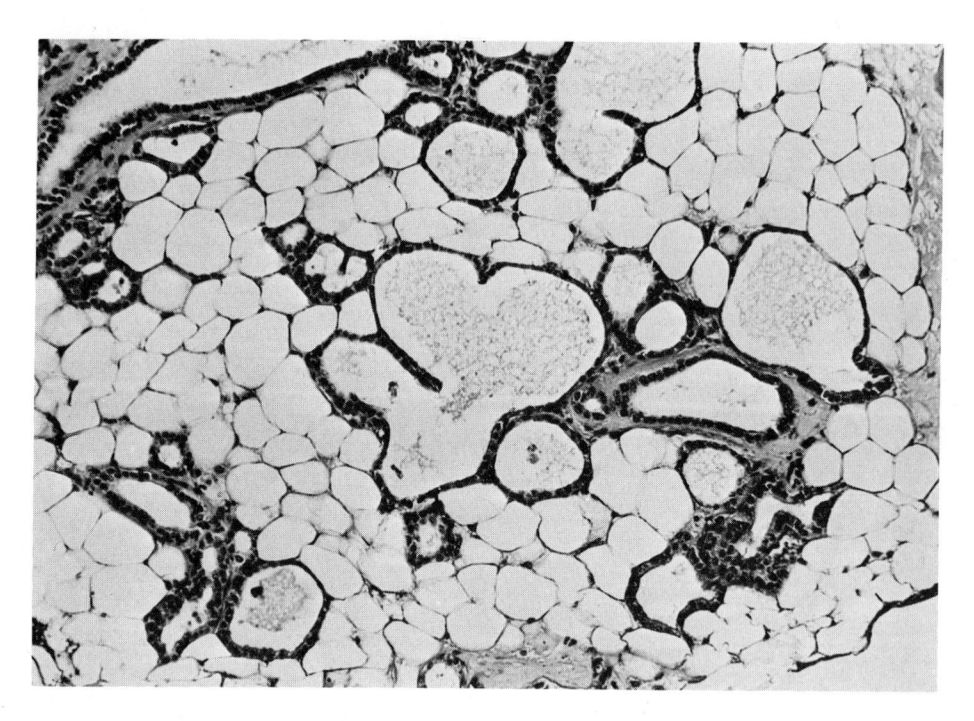

Figure 1. Mouse breast tissue after incubation in the absence of prolactin. Lumina of tubules are empty. x 150 (from Frantz, Kleinberg, and Noel, 1972).

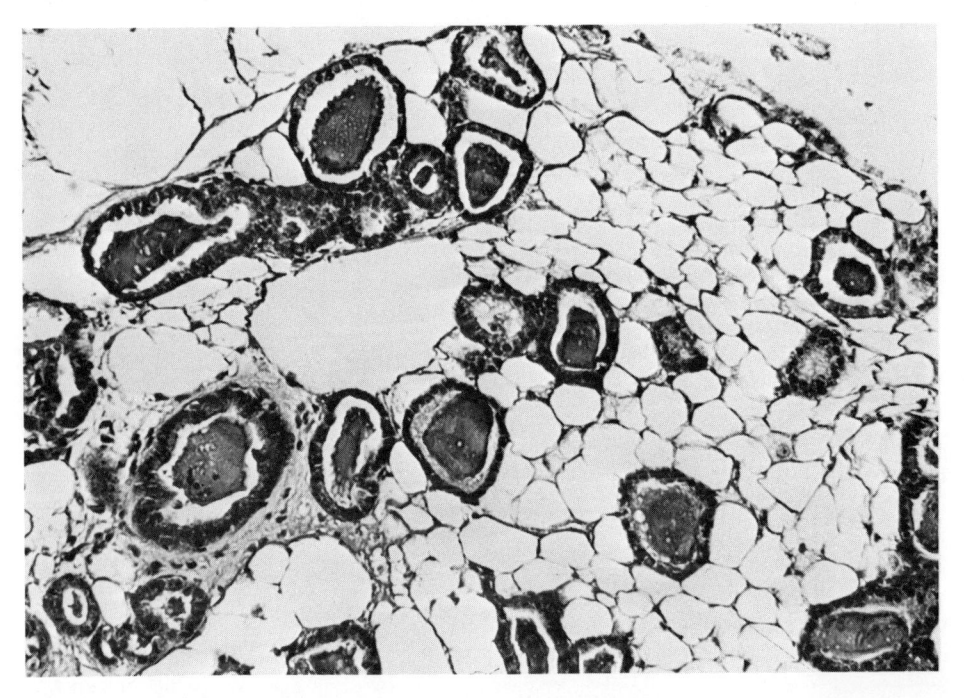

Figure 2. Mouse breast tissue after incubation in the presence of prolactin, 50 ng/ml. Lumina of tubules are filled with dark red-staining secretory material. x 150 (from Frantz et al., 1972).

arbitrarily graded on a scale of 0 to 4+, according to the number of lumina exhibiting secretory material, the degree of filling and also to some extent the depth of staining of the material. In practice this is not very difficult and the results of different observers are in good agreement. Intermediate responses between the fixed grades are possible since a mean is taken of the scores for each of the 3 or 4 fragments present in an incubation dish.

Figure 3 shows a composite curve based on a number of assays, in the majority of which 5 ng/ml is clearly distinguishable from zero. Thus the assay did in fact prove to have a much higher sensitivity than existing bioassays. The precision of this assay is inherently low. Nevertheless it can be made to yield acceptable precision when a sample is assayed, as is always done, at more than one dilution, and in at least two or preferably three assays. Under these conditions we were able to obtain a coefficient of variation of 25%-35%, which was adequate for our work at that time. The specificity of the assay is high. Only known lactogens give positive responses and these include prolactin itself, human growth hormone,

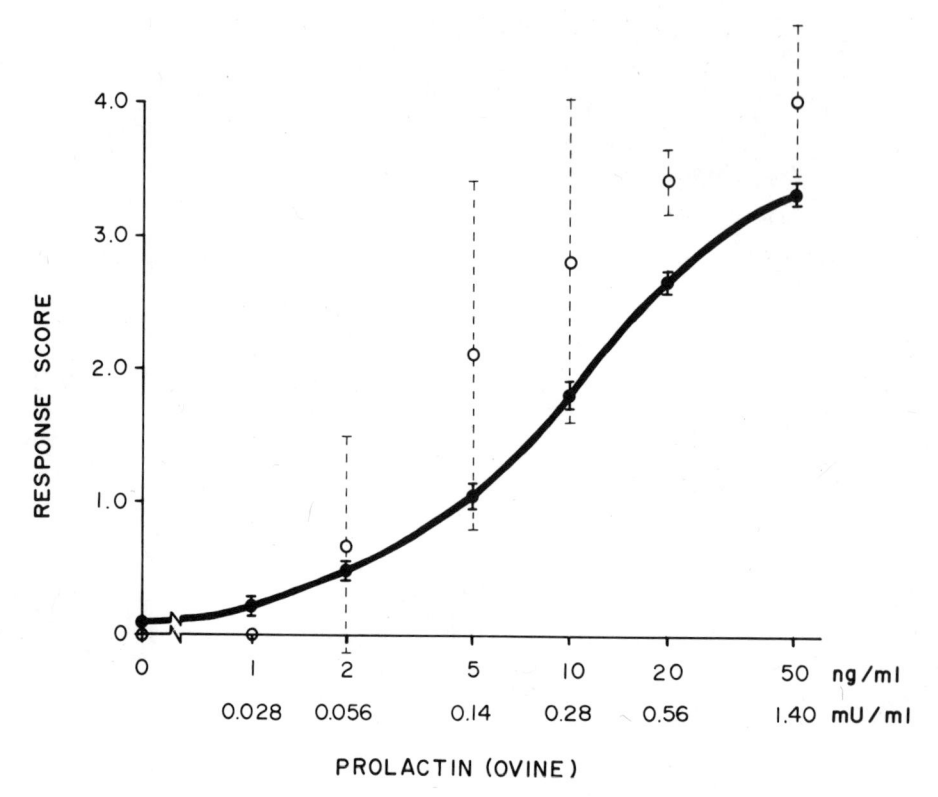

Figure 3. Standard dose response curve for ovine prolactin. Solid line and bars represent the mean of 60 assays, ± standard error of the mean. Open circles and dashed lines represent the responses derived from a single assay (from Frantz et al., 1972).

and human placental lactogen. Of the many other substances tested, including estrogens and progestins, none gave positive responses.

When this assay was applied to the study of human plasma it immediately became obvious that prolactin activity was present in a large number of plasma samples. It was almost always detectable in the blood of nursing mothers, in some patients with tumors, in some but by no means all patients with galactorrhea, and in patients on various drugs. Normal individuals, on the other hand, almost never had detectable prolactin activity, the threshold of the assay being approximately 15 ng/ml of ovine prolactin equivalents, this representing an average sensitivity of 5 ng/ml and a one-third dilution factor of the plasma. Human growth hormone itself is a potent lactogen, having an activity 50%-80% that of ovine prolactin, in this bioassay. If sufficiently elevated in plasma, as in most acromegalic plasmas, it will give a positive response. However, we were able to show that the prolactin activity of human growth hormone itself, whether the hormone was added exogenously to the medium or was present endogenously in acromegalic plasma could be completely neutralized by the addition of a potent anti-hGH antiserum. The same antiserum had no effect on the prolactin activity in the plasma of patients with galactorrhea or pituitary tumors. In some acromegalics, who were later shown to have elevated prolactin as well as hGH, neutralization was only partial. These results are shown graphically in Figure 4. It was clear, then, that we were dealing with a principle in human plasma which was separate from growth hormone and fulfilled all the criteria for a prolactin (Frantz and Kleinberg, 1970; Kleinberg and Frantz, 1971).

Two other mouse breast assays were reported shortly after this, one by Loewenstein and his colleagues in Daughaday's group (Loewenstein, Mariz, Peake, and Daughaday, 1971) and another by Turkington (1971), both using radiochemical endpoints. Essentially the same information was provided by these assays, which had the convenience of a completely objective endpoint. Because occasional samples may show signs of necrosis, and because occasionally a dish may contain fragments of tissue other than breast, there is some value in checking the histological appearance of the tissues in each dish. Whatever the endpoint, the precision remains inherently relatively low with this kind of an assay. The claim to precision of considerably less than 10% on interassay variation which Turkington reported (Turkington, 1971) we have not been able to reproduce, either by our assay or by Turkington's assay using his method.

Radioimmunoassay

The next advance in this field was the isolation of primate and human prolactin by two groups of investigators (Lewis, Singh, and Seavey, 1971; Hwang, Guyda, and Friesen, 1972). These provided source material for the development of homologous human radioimmunoassays which have since become the standard method of measuring the hormone (Hwang, Guyda, and Friesen, 1971; Sinha, Selby, Lewis, and VanderLaan, 1973). The studies of Jacobs and his colleagues had also shown that a heterologous assay based on an anti-ovine anti-serum and labelled porcine antigen could have the capability of measuring the hormone in human blood (Jacobs, Mariz, and Daughaday, 1972). Figure 5 shows the standard curve of a radioimmunoassay for the human hormone, using materials supplied by Dr. Henry Friesen. There is good sensitivity and no significant cross reaction by human growth hormone, even at amounts considerably greater than are shown in this figure. Any cross reactivity which exists can probably be ascribed to trace quantities of prolactin which contaminate the human growth hormone preparation. Figure 6 shows a number of samples assayed by both methods. We were encouraged

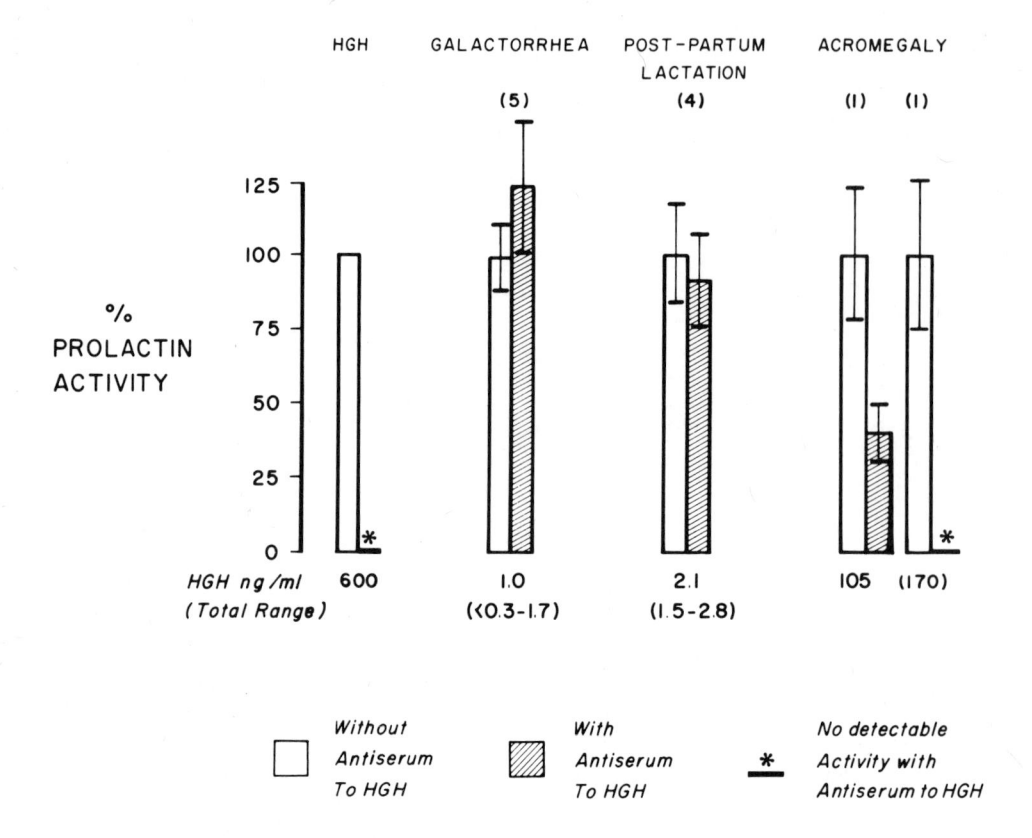

Figure 4. Prolactin activity of purified human growth hormone; also plasma samples from 5 patients with galactorrhea, 4 nursing mothers, and 2 patients with acromegaly. In each case samples were run with and without prior incubation of the sample with antiserum to human growth hormone. The level after incubation (shaded bars) is expressed as a per cent of the value before incubation (open bars), which is taken as 100%. Vertical lines indicate standard error of the mean (from Kleinberg and Frantz, 1971).

to find that the correlation was good at both the high and low ends of the range. Values less than 15 ng/ml, or unmeasurably low by the bioassay, were in the same range by radioimmunoassay; similarly, high values by bioassay came out high on the radioimmunoassay. The bioassay/radioimmunoassay potency ratio lay between 0.5 and 2.0

ASSAY AND REGULATION IN HUMANS 101

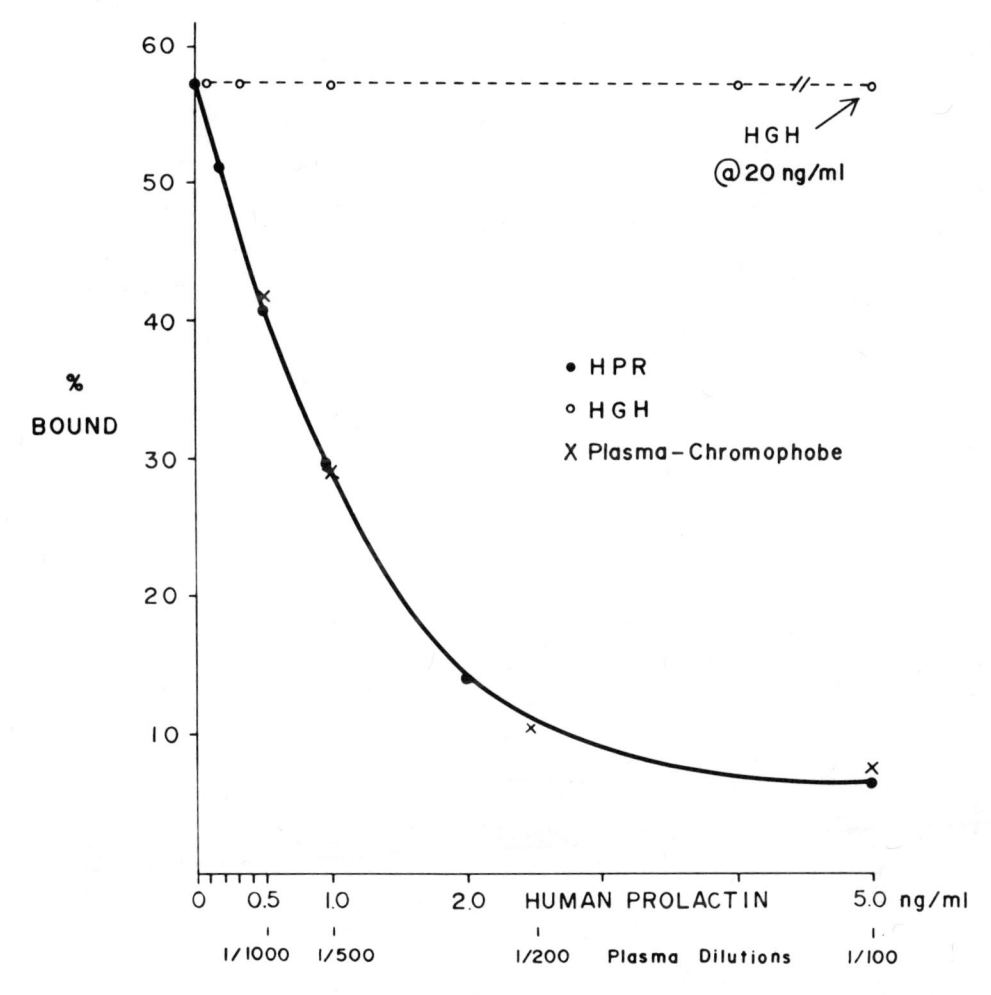

Figure 5. Standard curve of homologous radioimmunoassay using human prolactin standards and anti-human prolactin antibody. Plasma from a patient with a prolactin-secreting chromophobe adenoma yielded an identical curve when assayed at multiple dilutions (from Frantz et al., 1972).

in two-thirds of the samples which had measurable values by both assays, with a mean ratio of 1.09 (Frantz et al., 1972). This provides strong assurance that what is measured by the radioimmunoassay is indeed biologically active prolactin. We have encountered some plasma specimens where the ratio of the two activities is sufficiently different in either one direction or the other to suggest that in some patients there are molecules circulating which differ significantly from the normal hormone, either as a result of peri-

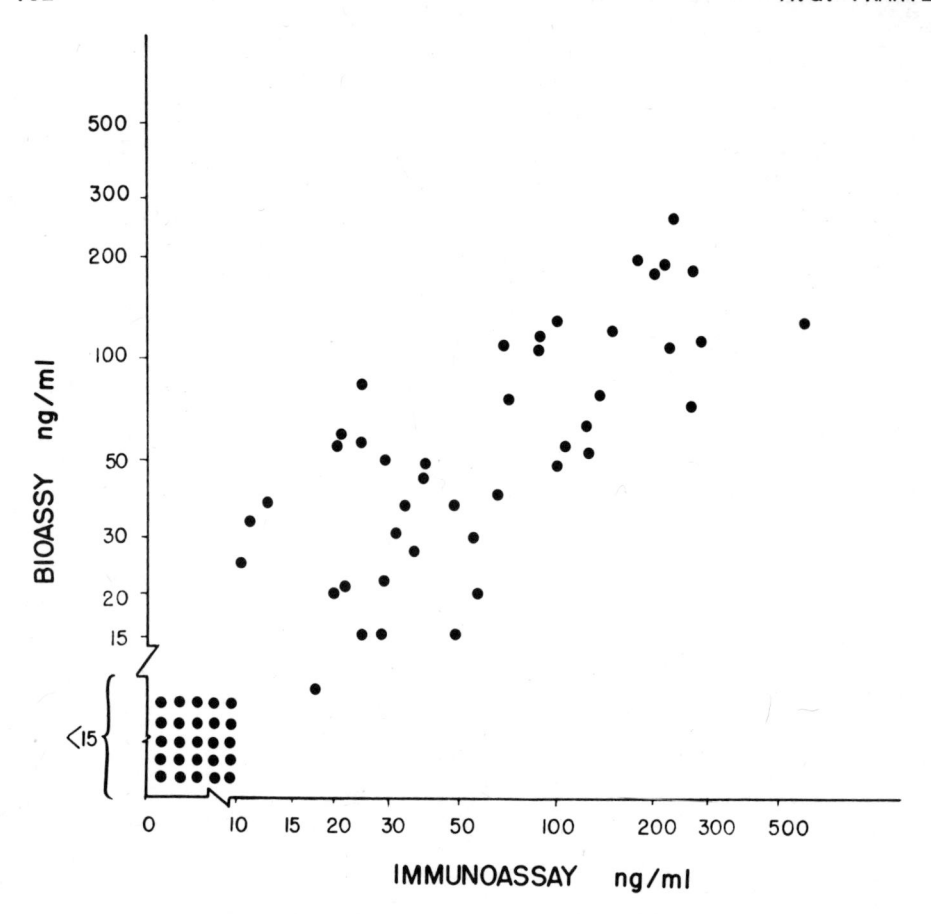

Figure 6. Correlation of bioassay and radioimmunoassay values on plasmas with varying concentrations of prolactin. Bioassay values were measured in terms of an ovine (NIH-P-S8), and radioimmunoassay in terms of a human (Friesen hPRL-71-9-4) standard (from Frantz et al., 1972).

pheral degradation or the secretion of some altered hormone.

Radioreceptor Assay

A recently reported development of considerable importance is the finding by Friesen and his colleagues of prolactin receptors in a number of tissues, including rabbit mammary tissue and rat liver. These appear to have specificity for lactogenic activity, in that human growth hormone is active in them while bovine growth hormone has little or no activity (Shiu, Kelly, and Friesen, 1973; Posner, Kelly, Shiu, and Friesen, 1974). Assays based on such

ASSAY AND REGULATION IN HUMANS   103

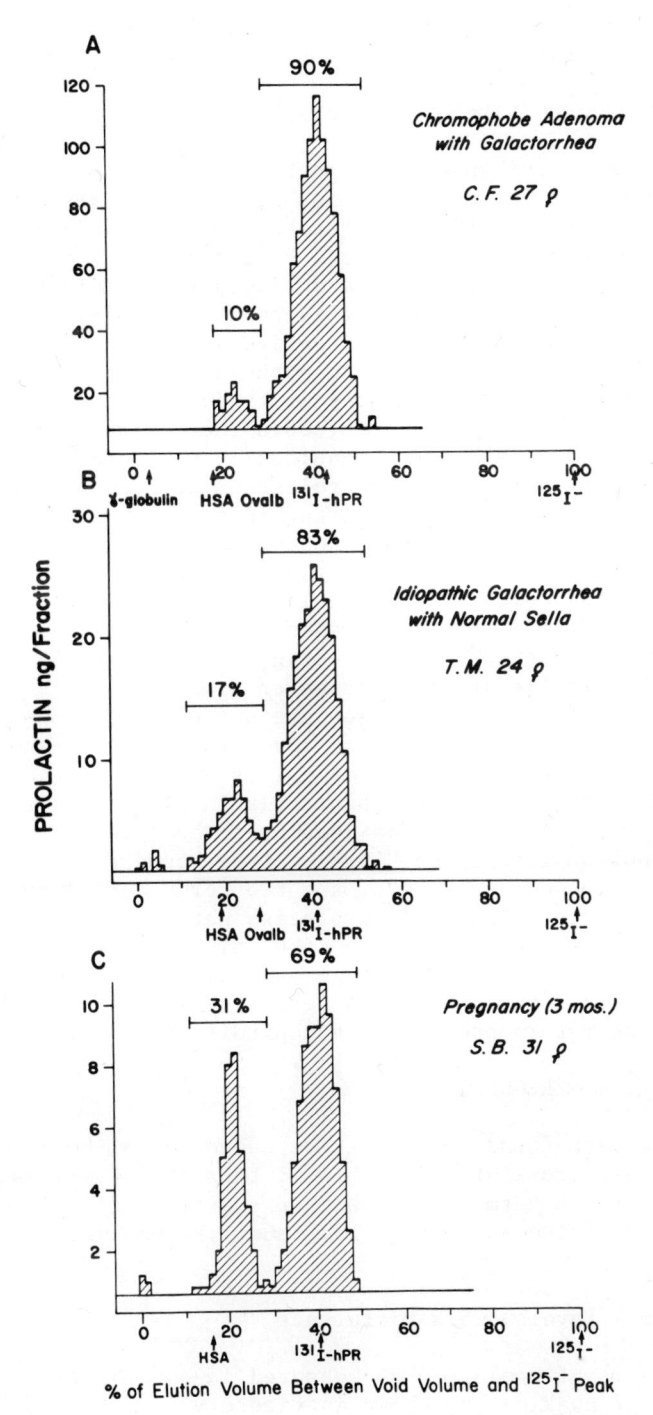

Figure 7.

Elution pattern of plasma samples from three different subjects, applied to 92 x 1.7 cm columns of Sephadex G-100. Volume of fractions was 2.0 ml. Mobility is expressed as a percentage of the effluent volume emerging between the void volume, determined with blue dextran, and the iodide-125 peak. HSA = human serum albumin tagged with bromphenol blue. Ovalb + Ovalb labeled with fluorescein. 131I-hPR = iodinated human prolactin reference standard (from Suh and Frantz, 1974).

receptors give promise of combining in some measure the specificity of bioassay with the convenience and precision of radioimmunoassay.

"Big" and "Little" Prolactin

Recently we have found evidence for size heterogeneity of circulating human prolactin similar to that which had been reported earlier for human growth hormone (Suh and Frantz, 1974). Similar findings have also been reported by Rogol and Rosen (1974). "Big" prolactin, eluting on Sephadex G-100 with a mobility suggesting a molecular size 2.5-3 times that of the highly purified prolactin standard--comprised 8%-31% of total immunoreactive prolactin in all plasma specimens examined, normal as well as pathological (Figure 7). Virtually all of the remaining immunoactivity in plasma eluted in a single peak, termed "little" prolactin, coincident with that of highly purified prolactin standard. Occasionally very small amounts of a third peak, termed "big big" prolactin, were found eluting close to the void volume. Major differences in the proportions of "big" and "little" prolactin have not been seen in the plasmas we have so far examined from patients with prolactin-secreting pituitary tumors as compared to normals. An exception to this appears to occur in normal pregnancy, when there is a distinct rise in the proportion of "big" prolactin. "Big" prolactin can be partly converted to the "little" form by repeated freezing and thawing or by prolonged frozen storage. We have not observed conversion of "little" to "big" prolactin under any circumstances, including incubation with hypopituitary plasma. This and the fact that we have seen small amounts of "big" prolactin in pituitary extracts and organ culture incubation media lead us to believe that "big" prolactin does not represent the "little" form bound to a plasma constituent. As shown in Figure 8, the two forms appear to be immunologically indistinguishable. The precise nature of the "big" form remains to be determined. Unlike the "big, big" form, which may increase in proportion with storage and which we believe may represent an aggregate, "big" prolactin seems to us more likely to represent a direct secretory product of the pituitary gland.

REGULATION

Many factors have been found to affect the secretion of human prolactin. Some of these are listed in Table 1; this also compares their action on human growth hormone, to which prolactin is chemically and biologically related (Niall, Hogan, Sauer, Rosenblum, and Greenwood, 1971).

Normal Levels. Sex Difference

Normal, adult levels of prolactin as measured in our laboratory several hours after awaking are shown in Figure 9. The

Table 1. SOME FACTORS AFFECTING PROLACTIN AND hGH SECRETION

	hPRL	hGH
Physiological:		
Sleep	↑↑	↑↑
Stress	↑↑	↑↑
Nursing	↑↑↑	N*
Breast stimulation (nonpostpartum)	↑	N
Hypoglycemia	↑	↑↑
Glucose	N	↓
Strenuous exercise	↑	↑
Sexual intercourse, women	↑	N
Pregnancy	↑↑↑	N
Estrogens	↑	↑
Hypothyroidism	↑	N
Pharmacological:		
Phenothiazines	↑↑	N or ↓
L-dopa	↓↓	↑↑
TRH	↑↑	N
Arginine	↑	↑↑
Ergot	↓↓	↑
Apomorphine	↓↓	↑↑
Somatostatin	N	↓

*N = no change

range for men is <1.0 to 20 ng/ml, with a mean of 4.72 ± 2.82 ng/ml (standard deviation). The range for women is 1-25 ng/ml with a mean of 8.00 ± 4.96 ng/ml. The sex difference is statistically significant ($\bar{p}$<0.001) in the 102 subjects studied, though the overlap in total range was very great for the two sexes. Prolactin concentrations in the newborn are high, declining by six weeks to the adult range (Hwang, Friesen, Hardy, and Wilansky, 1971). The adult sex difference in levels makes its appearance around the time of puberty (Ehara, Yen, and Siler, 1975).

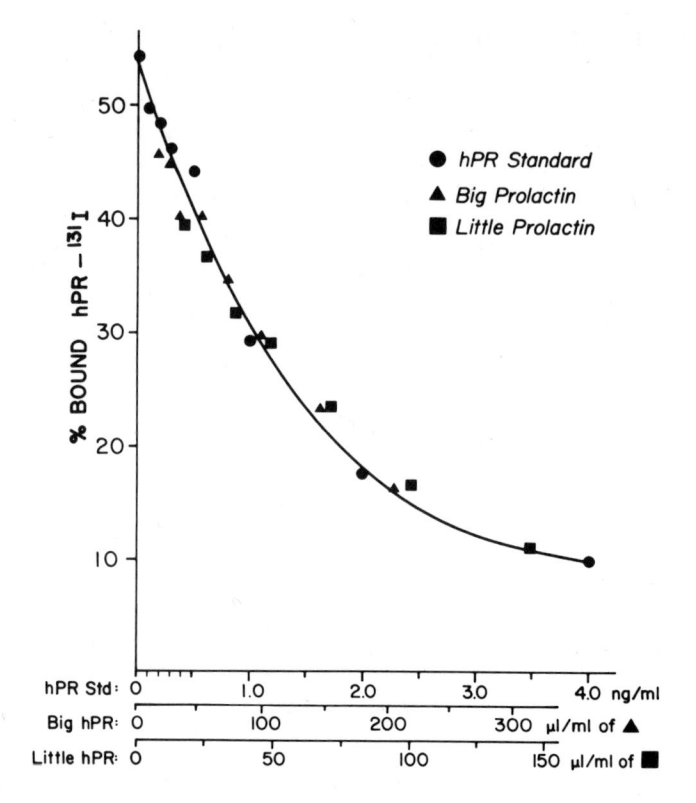

Figure 8. Radioimmunoassay of "big" and "little" prolactin fractions from plasma assayed at multiple dilutions, together with purified human prolactin standard (from Suh and Frantz, 1974).

Nursing and Breast Stimulation

As was first indicated by the animal studies of Reece and Turner (1937), nursing in women releases prolactin and may be the most specific and potent of all physiological prolactin-releasing stimuli in the human. Figure 10 shows the effect of a 30-minute nursing episode on plasma prolactin in women at various times postpartum. Prolactin rises rapidly after the beginning of suckling, reaching a maximum close to the end of the episode and declining thereafter to baseline levels (Noel, Suh, and Frantz, 1974). There is probably not a complete cessation of secretion with the termination of nursing, since the decline is a little slower than what other studies have shown to be the half-life of the hormone, i.e., 15-20 minutes. It is interesting that baseline levels of prolactin

ASSAY AND REGULATION IN HUMANS 107

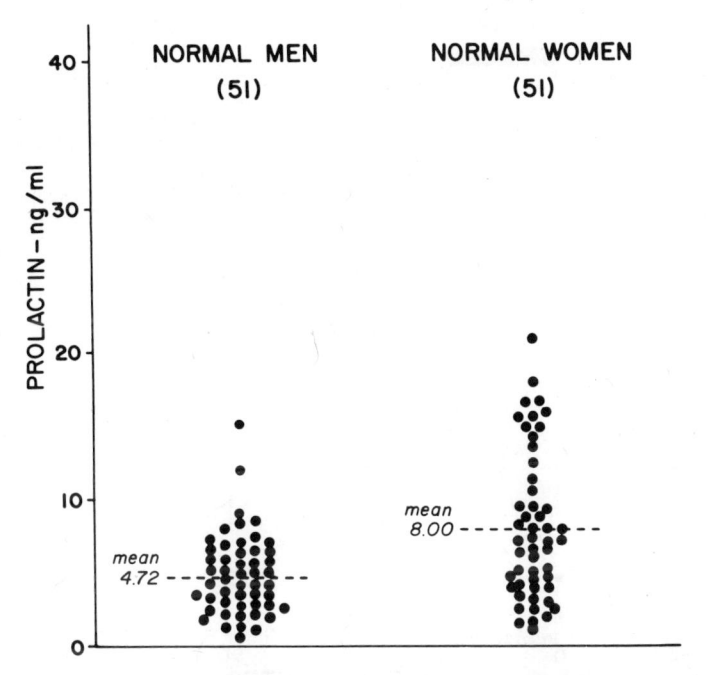

Figure 9. Plasma prolactin, measured by radioimmunoassay, in 51 normal men and 51 normal women, aged 18 to 67 years.

in lactating women many weeks post-partum may be well within the normal range, though we have always seen some response to the stimulus of nursing. These observations are similar to those of Tyson, Friesen, and Anderson (1972). That the stimulus is physical, rather than psychic, is indicated by the fact that anticipation of nursing without actual breast contact failed to cause prolactin release, even when milk let-down occurred; as it did in several of our patients during the period prior to nursing. Prolactin release of equal magnitude to that induced by nursing can also be caused in lactating women by the use of a breast pump (Noel *et al.*, 1974). Breast stimulation in normally menstruating, nonpost-partum women causes significant prolactin release in only about one-third of the subjects in our experience (Noel *et al.*, 1974). Men show no effect of breast stimulation on prolactin (Figure 11). Similar findings have been reported by Kolodny, Jacobs, and Daughaday (1972), except that these authors found prolactin release in all normal women studied after breast stimulation. It appears likely that the reflex to prolactin secretion by breast stimulation exists at least in latent form in all women, is greatly enhanced by the hormonal events of pregnancy and parturition, and diminishes rapidly thereafter.

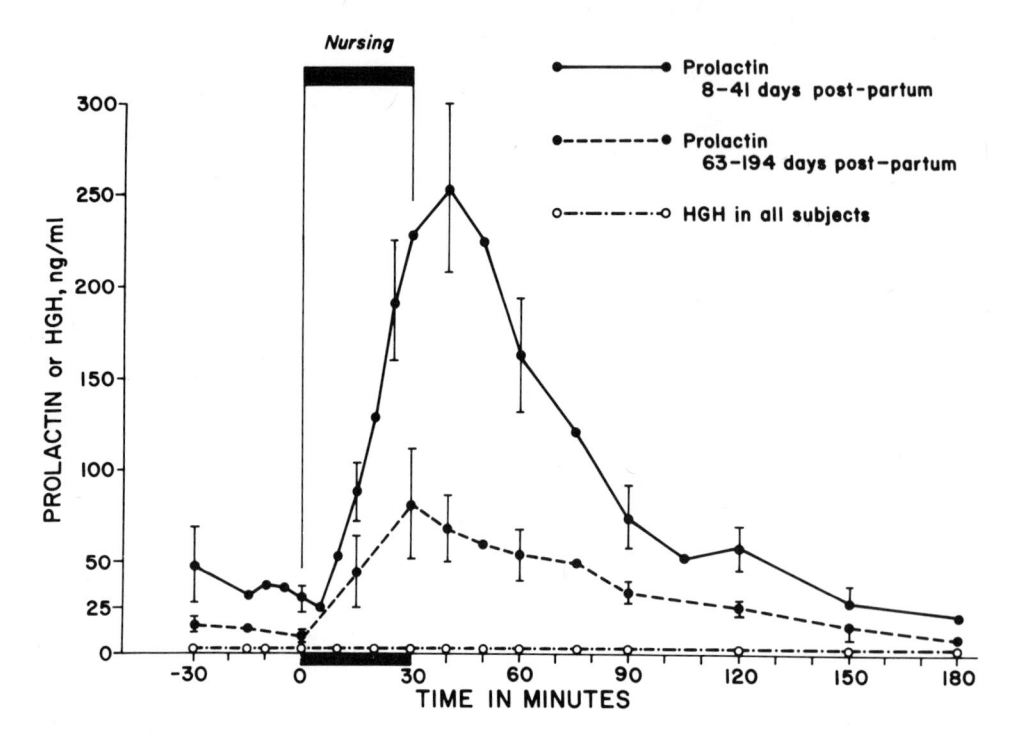

Figure 10. Plasma prolactin and growth hormone concentrations during nursing in post-partum women. Twelve studies were performed on 8 women between 8 and 41 days post-partum, and six studies on 6 women between 63 and 194 days post-partum. Vertical lines indicate standard error of the mean. Growth hormone, shown at the bottom, did not rise with suckling (from Noel et al., 1974).

24-hour Studies and the Effect of Sleep

A pronounced 24-hour variation in plasma production has been noted, based on samples taken every 20 minutes throughout the day and night (Sassin, Frantz, Weitzman, and Kapen, 1972). As shown in Figures 12 and 13, the highest levels occur at night, shortly after the onset of sleep. That the night-time peak is related to sleep itself, and not to an intrinsic 24-hour circadian rhythm, has been shown by sleep reversal studies, in which subjects were kept awake all night and allowed to go to sleep during the morning hours (Sassin, Frantz, Kapen, and Weitzman, 1973; Parker, Rossman, and VanderLaan, 1973). The sleep-associated prolactin rise differs both in time of onset and in duration from the night-time growth

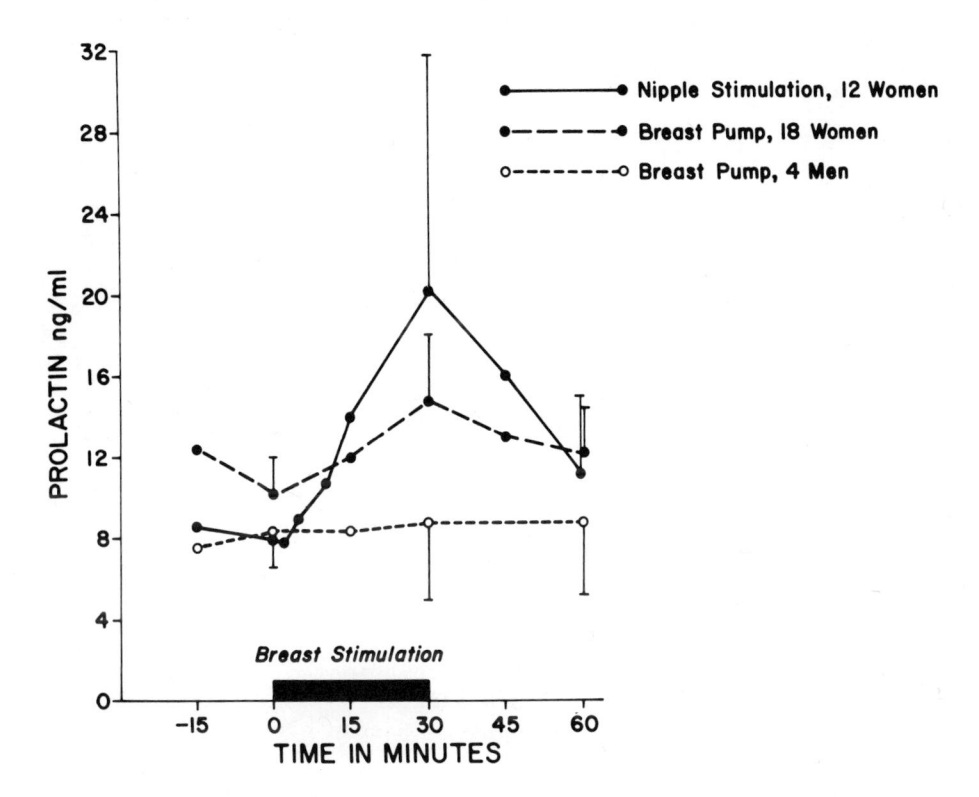

Figure 11. Effect of breast stimulation on plasma prolactin in normal nonpost-partum women and in men. Only 7 of the 18 women tested with the breast pump, and 2 of the 12 tested with manual stimulation of the breast and nipple, had significant prolactin rises (from Noel et al., 1974).

hormone rise, which is also associated with sleep (Takahashi, Kipnis, and Daughaday, 1968; Sassin, Parker, Mace, Gotlin, Johnson, and Rossman, 1969). Unlike the nocturnal growth hormone peak, that of prolactin cannot be correlated with a particular stage of the electroencephalogram. Though limited studies to date have indicated that the 24-hour variation in prolactin is usually abolished in patients with pituitary tumors as well as certain other disorders, we and others have noted that it is usually normal in those patients with galactorrhea who menstruate regularly (Malarkey, 1975; Kleinberg, Noel, and Frantz, 1976).

Stress

Stress of many kinds, particularly that due to major surgery with general anesthesia, is associated with rises in prolactin.

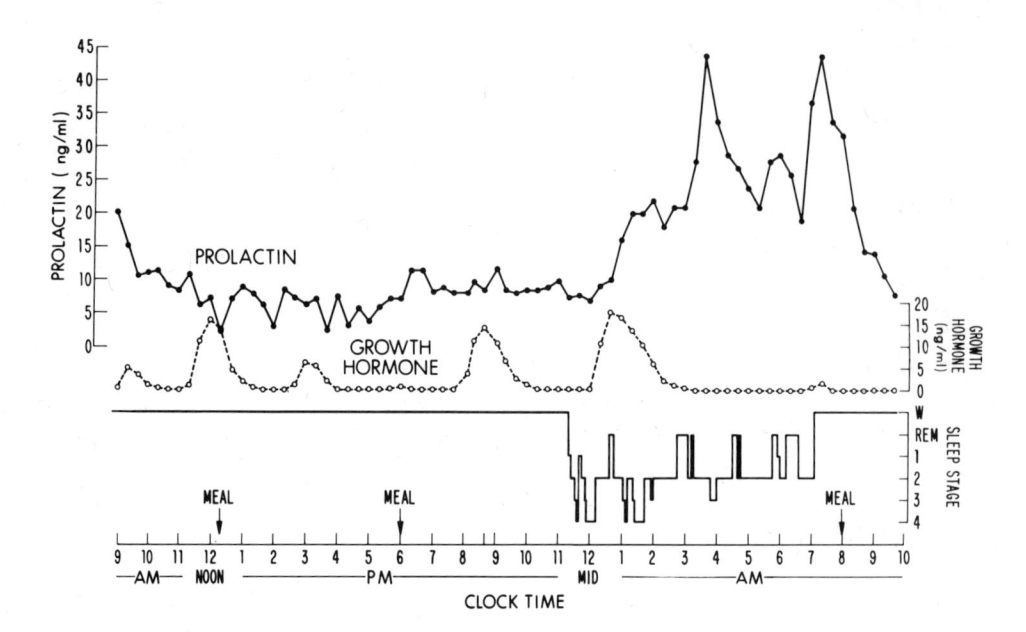

Figure 12. Plasma prolactin and growth hormone, measured at 20-minute intervals, in a single subject. Normal sleep was monitored by EEG (from Sassin et al., 1972).

These are usually at least equal in magnitude of those of growth hormone under similar circumstances, though in individual subjects the two hormones are not necessarily released at the same time or in similar relative amounts (Noel, Suh, Stone, and Frantz, 1972).

Hypoglycemia

Severe hypoglycemia, such as occurs during the course of insulin tolerance tests, may be associated with prolactin rises (Frantz et al., 1972; Noel et al., 1972; Copinchi, L'Hermite, Leclerq, Goldstein, Van Haelst, Virasoro, and Robyn, 1975). In our experience a greater degree of hypoglycemia is required to elicit a prolactin rise than is necessary to stimulate growth hormone, and insulin hypoglycemia is not a generally reliable test of prolactin pituitary reserve. Glucose administration causes little, if any, change in prolactin.

Exercise

Strenuous exercise has been observed to cause a prolactin rise, similar to but smaller than that of growth hormone under the same conditions (Noel et al., 1972).

ASSAY AND REGULATION IN HUMANS   111

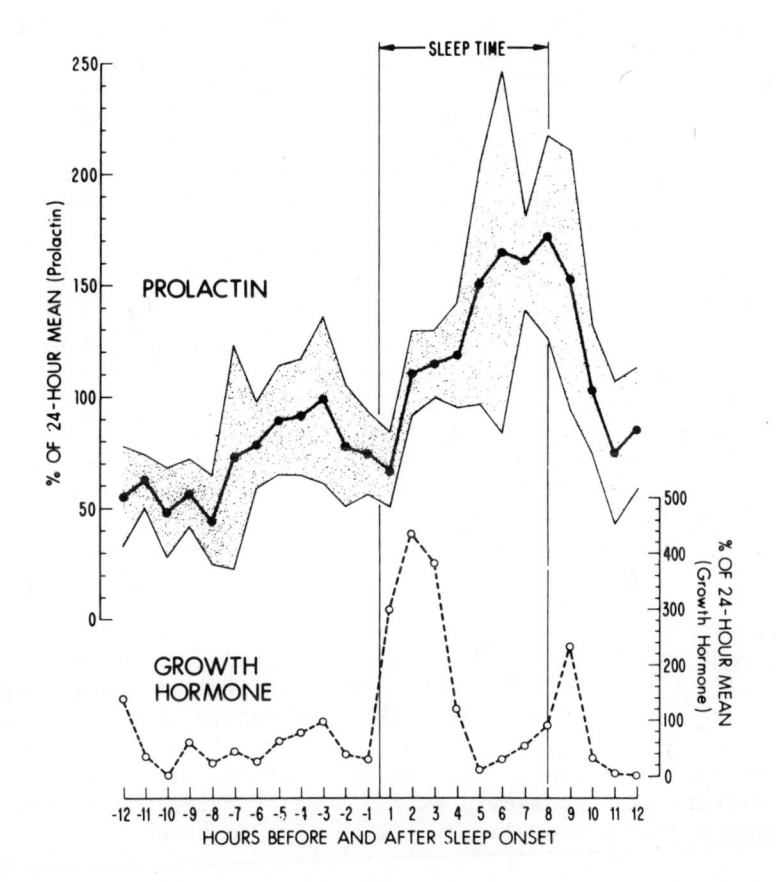

Figure 13. Prolactin and growth hormone in 6 normal subjects (3
            men and 3 women) measured under the same conditions as
            indicated for Figure 12. For clarity in the figure,
            three 20-minute values were averaged to give an hourly
            figure for each subject and the hourly results express-
            ed as a percentage of the 24-hour mean for that subject.
            Solid line represents mean prolactin at hourly inter-
            vals for all six subjects. Shaded area is ± 1 standard
            deviation (from Sassin *et al.*, 1972).

Sexual Intercourse

A marked rise in plasma prolactin has been noted in a minority of normal women following sexual intercourse. The rise occurred only in women who experienced orgasm. It was not related to or dependent on associated breast stimulation. No significant rise occurred in the male partners of these subjects. Human growth hormone did not change after sexual intercourse in either sex (Noel et al., 1972). Those findings have been confirmed (Stearns, Winter, and Faiman, 1973). It is unclear how these prolactin changes, the first of any hormonal changes to be observed in the human after sexual intercourse, relate to the other stimuli which have been associated with prolactin release.

Changes in Osmolality

Animal work has indicated an osmoregulator role for prolactin in certain species, the hormone generally acting to conserve sodium and to facilitate the transition from a more saline to a less saline environment. An effect of sudden changes in plasma osmolality on prolactin in humans was reported by Buckman and colleagues (Buckman and Peake, 1973a; Buckman, Kaminsky, Conway, and Peake, 1973), in which, somewhat paradoxically, hypotonic saline and water loading were found to suppress, and hypertonic saline to increase, plasma levels of the hormone. We have repeated these studies in our own laboratory, using considerably more subjects and a homologous rather than a heterologous radioimmunoassay, and have been unable to confirm Buckman's findings. If anything, there appeared to be a slight rise, rather than a fall, in prolactin with hypotonic saline (Adler, Noel, Wartofsky, and Frantz, 1975). Though further studies involving the administration of purified human prolactin, when available, will be of interest, it presently seems to us unlikely that prolactin exerts a major role in the short-term regulation of water and electrolyte balance in humans.

Pregnancy

A progressive rise in plasma prolactin takes place during the course of normal pregnancy (Hwang et al., 1971; L'Hermite and Robyn, 1972). It has been speculated that this phenomenon may be due to high circulating estrogen levels in the human, since in the monkey, where estrogen production during pregnancy is much lower, a comparable prolactin rise does not occur (Hwang et al., 1971).

Estrogens

A rise in plasma prolactin after the administration of large doses of estrogens in humans has been observed (Frantz et al., 1972; Yen, Ehara, and Siler, 1974). The main effect of estrogen appears to be more to sensitize the hypothalamic-pituitary axis to prolactin-releasing stimuli of various kinds than to raise resting levels of the hormone (Buckman and Peake, 1973b; Carlson, Jacobs, and Daughaday, 1973). A similar sensitizing action of estrogen on the mechanisms for releasing growth hormone was first noted by Frantz and Rabkin (1965). It seems likely that the greater responsiveness of women than men to almost all prolactin-releasing stimuli can be accounted for by their higher circulating levels of estrogen. Interestingly, an effect of the menstrual cycle on plasma prolactin levels has not been definitely corroborated in humans. Two groups of investigators have reported no change during the menstrual cycle (Hwang et al., 1971; McNeilly, Evans, and Chard, 1973), whereas a third group observed a rise at mid-cycle and during the luteal phase (Vekemans, Delvove, L'Hermite, and Robyn, 1972).

Thyroid Hormones

A relationship between thyroid hormone and prolactin secretion was suggested a number of years ago by clinical observations that galactorrhea is a rare complication of hypothyroidism, both in adults and children, in whom it may be associated with precocious puberty (Van Wyk and Grumbach, 1960). More recently it has been observed that prolactin may be elevated in some patients with myxedema, particularly those with galactorrhea, whose levels may diminish following treatment (Edwards, Forsyth, and Besser, 1971). Although baseline prolactin concentrations are within the normal range in the majority of patients with hypothyroidism, responsiveness to most prolactin-releasing stimuli is enhanced in these patients. Hypothyroidism increases, and hyperthyroidism or the administration of thyroid hormone decreases, prolactin responsiveness. The effects of altered thyroid function on prolactin are less marked, however, than are those on TSH (Bowers, Friesen, Hwang, Guyda, and Folkers, 1971; Snyder, Jacobs, Utiger, and Daughaday, 1973). The relationship between prolactin secretion and that of TSH is still unclear. In spite of the common action of TRH on both hormones (see below), there is much physiological evidence and some data from direct measurement to indicate that the two hormones are by no means generally secreted together. Thus, TSH is not released by the stimuli either of nursing (Gautvik, Weintraub, Graeber, Maloof, Zuckerman, and Tashjian, 1973) or of sexual intercourse (Stearns et al., 1973), nor is there a TSH rise in sleep parallel to that of prolactin.

TRH

TRH added to cloned pituitary cells *in vitro* was found to stimulate prolactin secretion (Tashjian, Barowsky, and Jensen, 1971), and it was later shown that TRH stimulated prolactin release in humans (Bowers et al., 1971; Jacobs, Snyder, Wilber, Utiger, and Daughaday, 1971). TRH, which can be presumed to act directly on the pituitary (though a hypothalamic site of action is not excluded), is thus a useful clinical test of pituitary prolactin responsiveness and/or secretory capacity. Studies in this laboratory have indicated that the prolactin content of the average human pituitary is relatively low compared to that of growth hormone, of the order of 100-200 µg/gland. Since the half-life of the hormone in blood is similar to that of growth hormone, i.e. 15-20 minutes, it is clear that the hormone has a relatively high turnover rate, and that a single injection of TRH may liberate more prolactin into the blood over a short period of time than is initially present in the gland. Thus TRH stimulates synthesis as well as release of prolactin, *in vivo* as well as *in vitro*.

The question of the role of TRH, if any, in the normal regulation of prolactin secretion is still uncertain. Limited studies with bolus injections of TRH have generally indicated that the smallest dose which releases TSH also releases prolactin (Jacobs, Snyder, Utiger, and Daughaday, 1973; Bowers, Friesen, and Folkers, 1973). Recently we studied the effects of prolonged TRH infusions in normal volunteers, beginning at sub-threshold concentrations and increasing gradually in stepwise increments. As shown in Figure 14, prolactin elevations began to be noticed at least as soon as those of TSH (Noel, Dimond, Wartofsky, Earll, and Frantz, 1974). TRH may, therefore, have a role in modulating prolactin secretion, though it would seem that sudden surges of prolactin secretion which are unaccompanied by TSH rises, such as those seen in nursing, are most likely to be caused by other mechanisms. These could be either abrupt decreases in prolactin inhibiting factor (PIF), or surges of some prolactin-releasing factor other than TRH. Evidence for the existence of one or more such factors has been obtained (Nicoll, Fiorindo, McKennee, and Parsons, 1970; Valverde, Chieffo, and Reichlin, 1972). It is also conceivable, though less likely, that there could be a sudden release of TRH accompanied by a simultaneous release of some as yet unidentified specific TSH-inhibiting factor.

Dopaminergic Control of Prolactin: Phenothiazines, L-dopa, and Related Drugs

The concept that prolactin is predominantly regulated by hypothalamic inhibition, through the secretion of PIF, has been solidly established by animal studies. It is also evident that PIF is, to a large extent, under dopaminergic control. Drugs such as the phenothiazines, which antagonize dopaminergic impulses, have been shown to elevate prolactin when given acutely, presumably by turning off PIF, as shown in Figure 15. These drugs thus constitute a test of hypothalamic as well as pituitary function (Kleinberg, Noel, and Frantz, 1971; Friesen, Guyda, Hwang, Tyson, and Barbeau, 1972). Prolactin determination may also serve as a useful objective measurement of the central nervous system effects of certain tranquilizers and other psychoactive drugs (Frantz and Sachar, 1976). L-dopa, given orally, inhibits prolactin release transiently in normal subjects, as shown in Figure 16; it is also effective in many patients with pathologic hyperprolactinemia (Kleinberg *et*

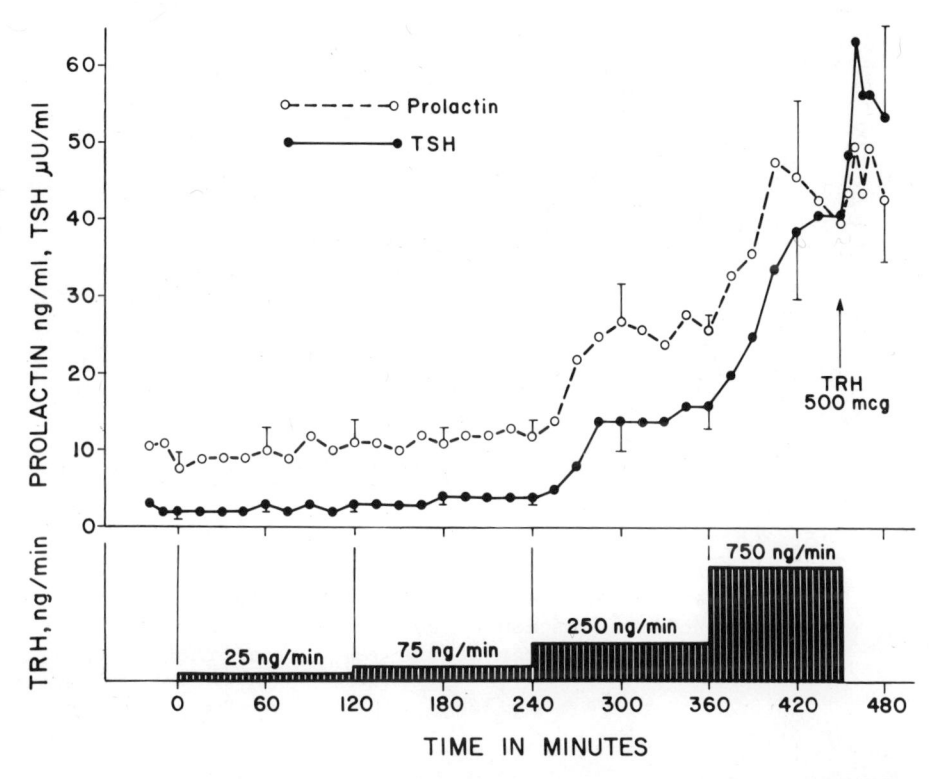

Figure 14. Prolactin and TSH responses to the continuous infusion of graded doses of TRH, followed by a 500 μg bolus of TRH, in 5 normal women. In this and other experiments, the smallest increases in TRH concentration capable of increasing plasma TSH also increased prolactin (from Noel et al., 1974).

al., 1971; Malarkey, Jacobs, and Daughaday, 1971; Friesen et al., 1972). As might be expected, L-dopa pretreatment can antagonize, for a time at least, the chlorpromazine-induced prolactin rise (Figure 17). A somewhat less expected result was the finding that L-dopa could also antagonize the rise of prolactin after TRH (Figure 18). This raises, but does not resolve, the question of where dopamine--the active metabolite to which L-dopa is converted after crossing the blood-brain barrier--is acting. Although there is definite evidence that dopamine can inhibit prolactin secretion by pituitaries cultivated *in vitro*, the bulk of evidence has favored a primarily hypothalamic site of action for the drug. In recent studies, however, we have observed significant inhibition of prolactin secretion after L-dopa administration in rhesus monkeys who had undergone complete transection of the pituitary stalk with in-

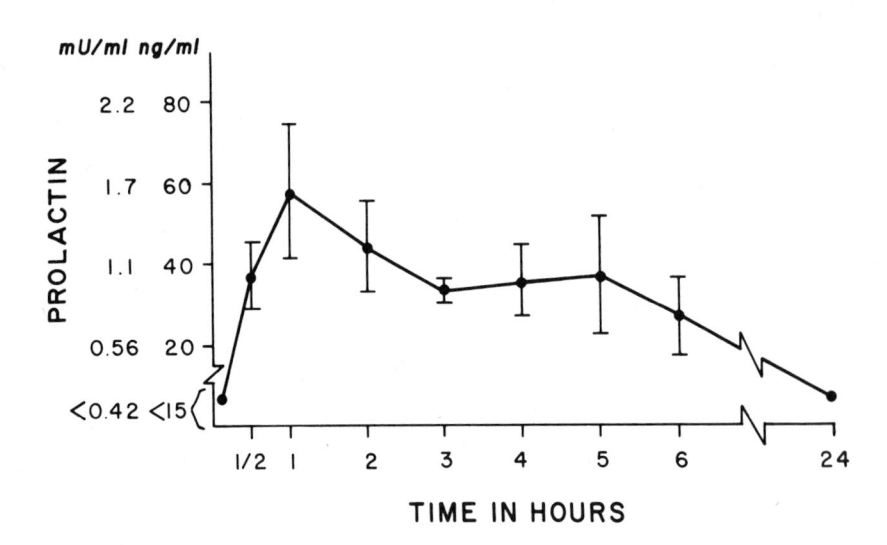

Figure 15. Chlorpromazine effect on plasma prolactin, studied in 9 normal subjects who received 25 mg chlorpromazine intramuscularly at the beginning of the experiment. Prolactin was measured by bioassay. Vertical bars denote standard error of the mean (from Frantz, 1973).

terposition of a silastic barrier, giving strong evidence that dopamine can act directly on the pituitary *in vivo* (Diefenbach, Carmel, Frantz, and Ferin, 1976).

Apomorphine, a dopamine analogue, suppresses prolactin transiently in humans (Lal, De La Vega, Sourkes, and Friesen, 1973). Ergot preparations have been shown to suppress prolactin in animals and two derivatives, 2-bromo-α-ergocryptine (Bromocriptin, CB-154, Sandoz), and Lergotrile (compound 83636, Lilly), have been shown to lower prolactin in humans and to be effective clinically in suppressing both puerperal and non-puerperal galactorrhea (del Pozo, Varga, Wyss, Tolis, Friesen, Wenner, Vetter, and Uettwiler, 1974; Lemberger, Crabtree, Clemens, Dyke, and Woodburn, 1974; Cleary, Crabtree, and Lemberger, 1975). The mechanism of action of ergot preparations appears to be principally directly on the pituitary, though a hypothalamic action is not ruled out. The superiority of ergot preparations to L-dopa as prolactin suppressants in the human is due at least in part to their longer duration of action. L-dopa may be effective as treatment in an occasional patient with galactorrhea, but in general does not seem to achieve sufficiently complete or

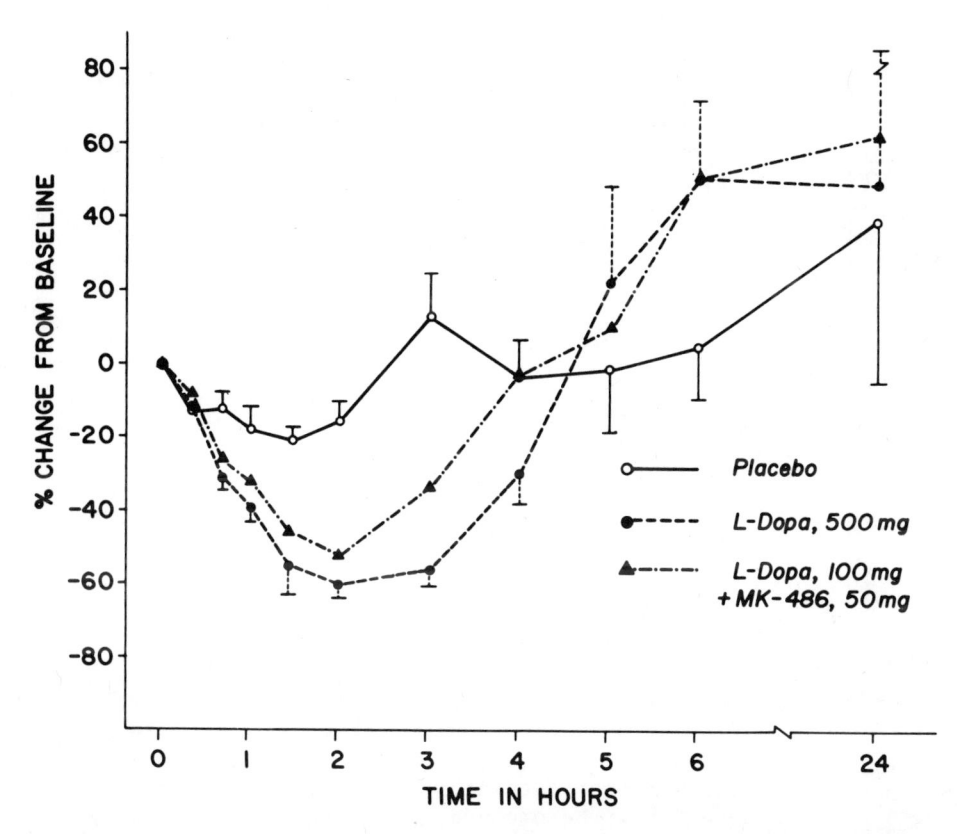

Figure 16. Plasma prolactin after a single oral dose of L-dopa, 500 mg, or L-dopa, 100 mg + MK-486, 50 mg (an inhibitor of peripheral decarboxylation of L-dopa), given at 0 time. All studies were done in 6 normal volunteers (3 men, 3 women) on different occasions. The response to an identically packaged placebo is also shown (from Frantz, Suh, and Noel, 1973).

prolonged suppression when given in usual dose schedules to be useful. An attempt to induce remission of breast cancer by suppressing prolactin secretion with L-dopa led to a small number of transient remissions, in our experience (Frantz, Habif, Hyman, Suh, Sassin, Zimmerman, Noel, and Kleinberg, 1973). Doses were given at frequent intervals, but the extent of suppression of 24-hour secretion could not be adequately assessed. Preliminary results with CB-154 used for this same purpose in patients with breast

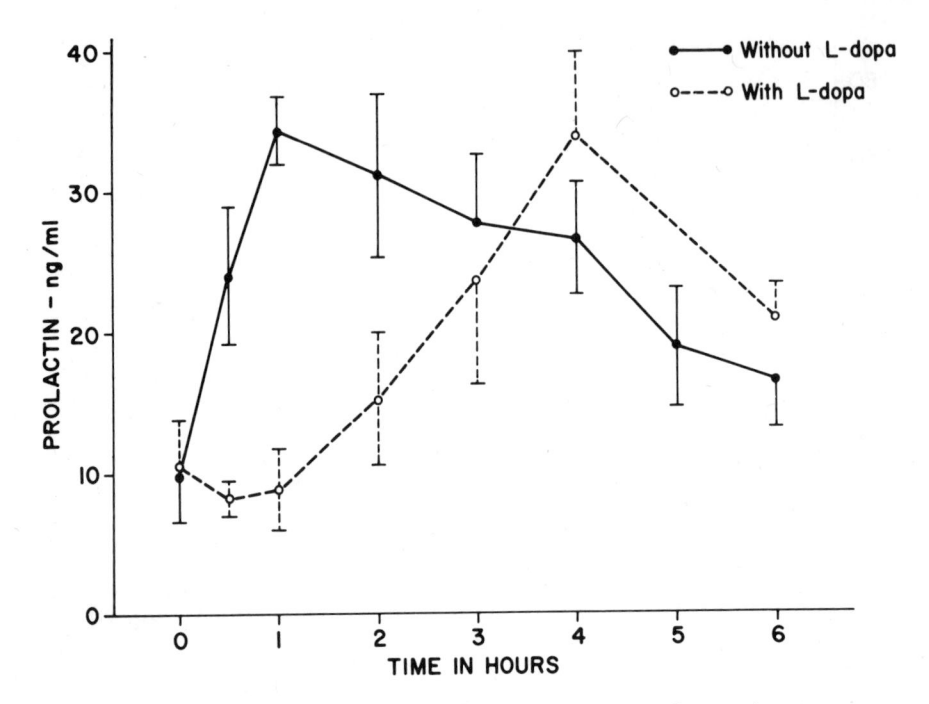

Figure 17. Plasma prolactin in four subjects after the intramuscular injection of 25 mg of chlorpromazine (solid line), and again on a subsequent occasion in the same individuals after pretreatment with 500 mg of L-dopa orally one-half hour beforehand (dashed line). Marked inhibition of the chlorpromazine-induced response is seen for the first two hours; after this suppression wanes because of the much shorter duration of action of L-dopa as compared with chlorpromazine.

cancer unfortunately have not been encouraging (Heuson, Coune, and Staquet, 1972).

Pathological States

A detailed discussion of clinical disorders of prolactin se-

Figure 18. Prolactin response to intravenous TRH given at 0 time in 7 normal women (top figure) and 7 normal men (bottom figure). Solid lines represent response to TRH alone: dashed lines represent same subjects tested again on a subsequent occasion after pretreatment with 500 or 750 mg of L-dopa orally at -60 minutes. A clear inhibition by L-dopa is evident (from Noel, Suh, and Frantz, 1973).

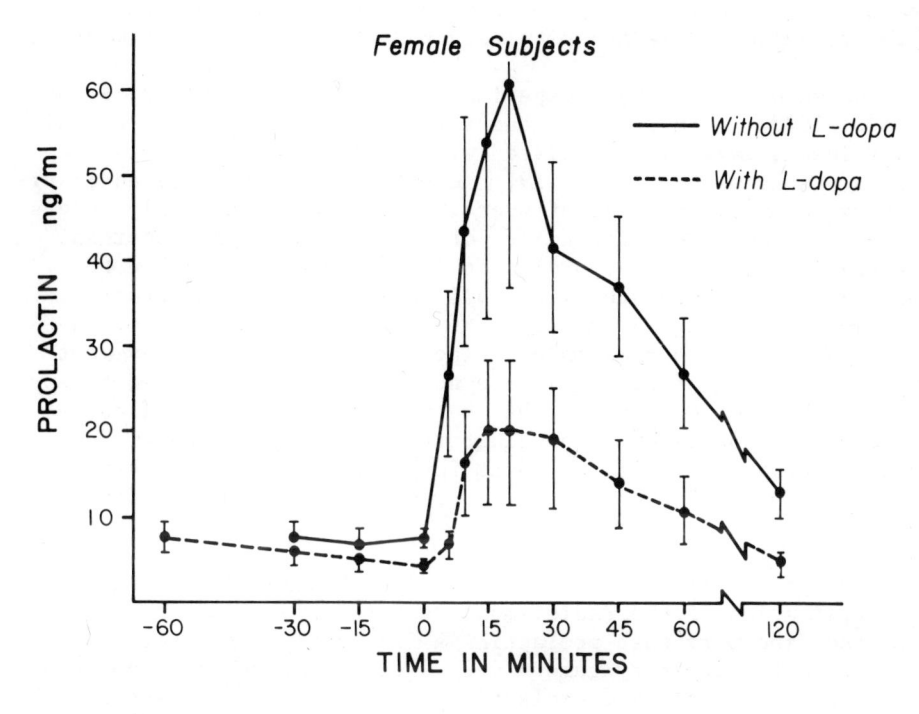

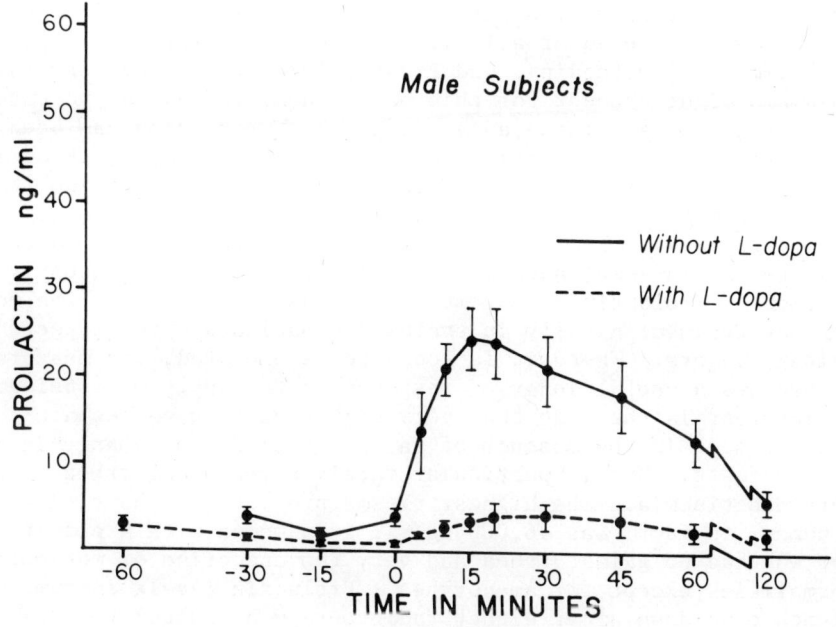

Figure 18

cretion is beyond the scope of the present paper. Two conditions, however, galactorrhea and pituitary tumors, deserve brief mention.

Galactorrhea, in our experience (Frantz *et al.*, 1972; Frantz *et al.*, 1973) as in that of others (Tolis, Somma, Van Campenhout, and Friesen, 1974) is associated with a wide range of prolactin values. As shown in figure 19, the highest are encountered in pituitary tumors, any value of over 200 ng/ml being strongly suggestive of a tumor. A large number of patients with galactorrhea, interestingly, will have prolactin levels which are within the normal range. Those are almost all patients whose galactorrhea is associated wtih regular menses, the largest single group of patients with galactorrhea in our experience. It is thus evident that high levels of prolactin are not necessarily required to sustain milk secretion, once it has been initiated. A detailed review of our experience with galactorrhea, including the use of suppression and stimulation tests for diagnosis and the results of different forms of therapy, is in preparation (Kleinberg *et al.*, 1976).

One of the most interesting clinical findings to emerge from the application of the radioimmunoassay for prolactin in humans has been the discovery that prolactin is frequently hypersecreted in patients with pituitary tumors even when galactorrhea is not present. In our experience, prolactin is elevated in at least one-third of all patients with chromophobe adenomas, making it the most commonly hypersecreted of all pituitary hormones (Frantz *et al.*, 1973; Zimmerman, Defendini, and Frantz, 1974). Although several mechanisms might account for this phenomenon, including increased secretion by normal tissue adjacent to the tumor which has been freed from hypothalamic inhibition by pressure on the stalk or its connections, immunocytochemical studies have suggested to us that it is the tumor itself which is hypersecreting the hormone (Zimmerman *et al.*, 1974). Lack of responsiveness to TRH in many cases, and to L-dopa in some, suggest that the secretion is frequently autonomous. Prolactin measurement has thus become one of the most important tests clinically in evaluating patients with suspected pituitary tumors. Where it is found to be elevated, its measurement becomes a useful index of response to therapy. Of considerable interest is the fact that very high prolactin values are sometimes seen in the absence of galactorrhea or any change in size of the breasts. Men in particular rarely have galactorrhea with hyperprolactinemia. The highest plasma prolactin we have seen in the human, in fact, was 46,000 ng/ml, in a woman with a pituitary tumor who had no galactorrhea and very few endocrine or metabolic abnormalities except for amenorrhea. Prolactin levels in tumor patients come down after either radiotherapy or surgery. Like growth hormone levels in patients with acromegaly, the decline after radiotherapy tends to be rather slow but progressive with time. Also, like growth hormone in acromegaly, prolactin in tumor

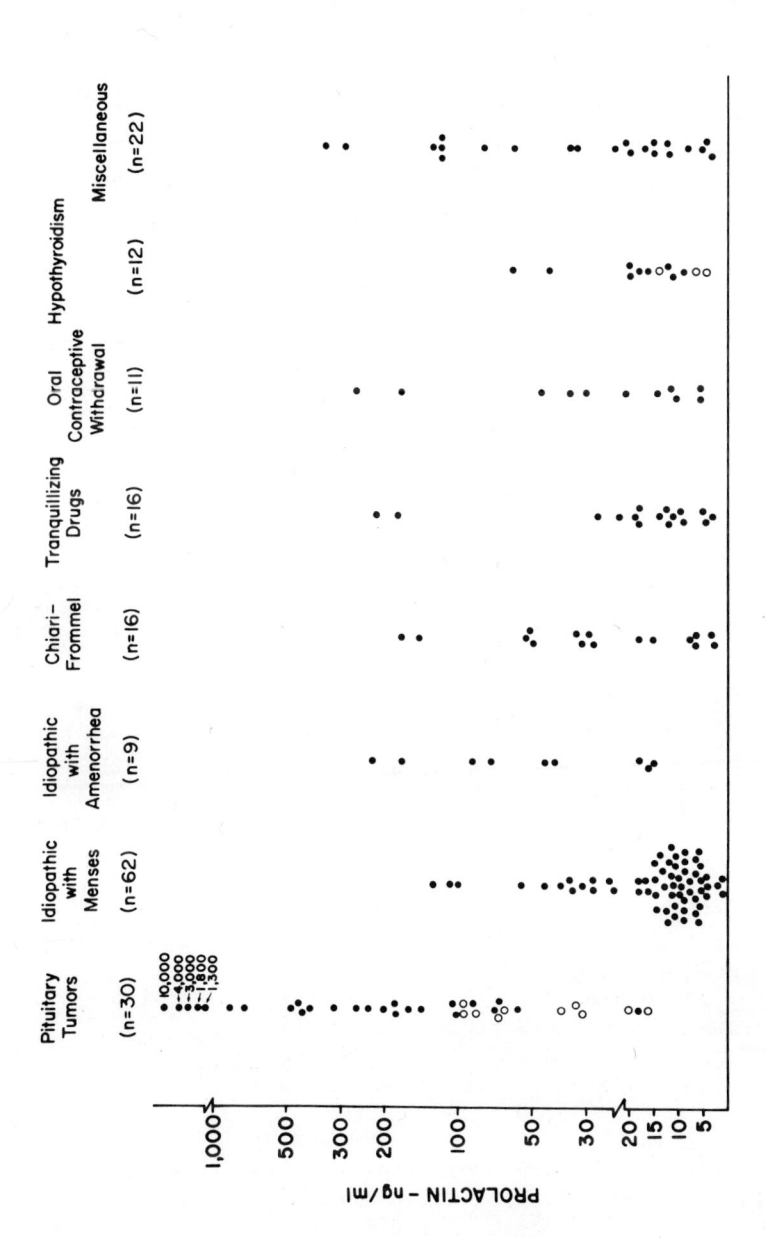

Figure 19. Plasma prolactin in 178 patients with galactorrhea of varying etiology. The highest levels, as a group, are seen in patients with pituitary tumors; the lowest most often within the normal range (1-25 ng/ml), in patients with idiopathic amenorrhea and regular menses. Open circles denote the tumor patients after treatment with surgery or radiotherapy.

patients most often does not come down all the way to normal, either after radiotherapy or transsphenoidal surgery. Hyperprolactinemia accompanies increased growth hormone secretion in 30%-40% of patients with acromegaly (Frantz *et al.*, 1972). Specific immunochemical stains on tumor specimens removed at surgery indicate that the two hormones are usually present in different cells. Nevertheless there is evidence that some cells in the normal pituitary may have the capability of secreting both hormones together (Zimmerman *et al.*, 1974).

In summary, the identification of human prolactin as a separate hormone and the development of assay techniques over the last five years have opened a new chapter in human pituitary physiology. Though as yet it is not clear what the functional role of the hormone is under many conditions, it can be expected that some of these questions may be answered when greater supplies of the hormone are available and it can be administered to humans for metabolic studies. Meanwhile its measurement will continue to provide valuable basic as well as clinical information concerning neuroendocrine control mechanisms in man.

REFERENCES

Adler, R.A., Noel, G.L., Wartofsky, L., and Frantz, A.G. (1975). Failure of oral water loading and intravenous hypotonic saline to suppress plasma prolactin in man. J. Clin. Endocrinol. Metab. 41, 383-389.

Bowers, C.Y., Friesen, H.G., and Folkers, K. (1973). Further evidence that TRH is also a physiological regulator of PRL secretion in man. Biochem. Biophys, Res. Comm. 51, 512-521.

Bowers, C.Y., Friesen, H.G., Hwang, P., Guyda, H.J., and Folkers, K. (1971). Prolactin and thyrotropin release in man by synthetic pyroglutamyl-histidyl-prolinamide. Biochem. Biophys. Res. Comm. 45, 1033-1041.

Buckman, M.T., Kaminsky, N., Conway, M., and Peake, G.T. (1973). Utility of L-dopa and water loading in evaluation of hyperprolactinemia. J. Clin. Endocrinol. Metab. 36, 911-919.

Buckman, M.T., and Peake, G.T. (1973a). Osmolar control of prolactin secretion in man. Science 181, 755-757.

Buckman, M.T., and Peake, G.T. (1973b). Estrogen potentiation of phenothiazine-induced prolactin secretion in man. J. Clin. Endocrinol. Metab. 36, 977-980.

Carlson, E.E., Jacobs, L.S., and Daughaday, W.H. (1973). Growth hormone, thyrotropin and prolactin responses to thyrotropin-releasing hormone following diethylstilbestrol pretreatment. J. Clin. Endocrinol. Metab. 37, 488-490.

Cleary, R.E., Crabtree, R., and Lemberger, L. (1975). The effect of lergotrile on galactorrhea and gonadotropin secretion. J. Clin. Endocrinol. Metab. 40, 830-833.

Copinschi, G., L'Hermite, M., Leclerq, R., Goldstein, J., Van Haelst, L., Virasoro, E., and Robyn, C. (1975). Effects of glucocorticoids on pituitary hormonal responses to hypoglycemia. Inhibition of prolactin release. J. Clin. Endocrinol. Metab. 40, 442-449.

DelPozo, E., Varga, L., Wyss, H., Tolis, G., Friesen, H., Wenner, R., Vetter, L., and Uettwiler, A. (1974). Clinical and hormonal response to bromocriptin (CB-154) in the galactorrhea syndromes. J. Clin. Endocrinol. Metab. 39, 18-26.

Diefenbach, R., Carmel, P.W., Frantz, A.G., and Ferin, M. (1976). Evidence for a direct action of L-dopa on the pituitary in rhesus monkeys. (Submitted for publication.)

Edwards, C.R.W., Forsyth, I.A., and Besser, G.M. (1971). Amenorrhoea, galactorrhoea, and primary hypothyroidism with high circulating levels of prolactin. Brit. Med. J. 3, 462-464.

Ehara, Y., Yen, S.S., and Siler, T.M. (1975). Serum prolactin levels during puberty. Amer. J. Obstet. Gynecol. 121, 995-997.

Elias, J.J. (1957). Cultivation of adult mouse mammary gland in hormone-enriched synthetic medium. Science 126, 824-844.

Frantz, A.G. (1973). Catecholamines and the control of prolactin secretion in humans. In: *Progress in Brain Research, Vol. 39. Drug Effects on Neuroendocrine Regulation* (Zimmerman, E., Gispen, W.H., Marks, B.H., and DeWied, D., eds.), pp. 311-321, Elsevier, Amsterdam.

Frantz, A.G., Habif, D.V., Hyman, G.A., Suh, H.K., Sassin, J.F., Zimmerman, E.A., Noel, G.L., and Kleinberg, D.L. (1973). Physiological and pharmacological factors affecting prolactin secretion, including its suppression by L-dopa in the treatment of breast cancer. In: *Human Prolactin* (Pasteels, J.L., and Robyn, C., eds.), pp. 273-290, Excerpta Medica, The Netherlands.

Frantz, A.G., and Kleinberg, D.L. (1970). Prolactin: Evidence that it is separate from growth hormone in human blood. Science 170, 745-749.

Frantz, A.G., Kleinberg, D.L., and Noel, G.L. (1972). Studies on prolactin in man. Recent Progr. Hormone Res. 28, 527-573.

Frantz, A.G., and Rabkin, M.T. (1965). Effects of estrogen and sex difference on secretion of human growth hormone. J. Clin. Endocrinol. Metab. 25, 1470-1480.

Frantz, A.G., and Sachar, E.J. (1976). Effects of antipsychotic drugs on prolactin and growth hormone levels in man. In: *Anti-Psychotic Drugs: Pharmacodynamics and Pharmacokinetics* (Sedvall, G., ed.), Karolinska Institute, Stockholm.

Frantz, A.G., and Suh, H.K. (1974). L-dopa and the control of prolactin secretion. In: *Advances in Neurology, Vol. 5* (McDowell, F.H., and Barbeau, A., eds.), pp. 447-456, Raven Press, New York.

Frantz, A.G., Suh, H.K., and Noel, G.L. (1973). Effects of L-dopa

on prolactin secretion in humans. In: *Frontiers in Catecholamine Research 1973* (Usdin, E., and Snyder, S., eds.), pp. 843-847, Pergamon Press, Great Britain.
Friesen, H., Guyda, H., Hwang, P., Tyson, J.E., and Barbeau, A. (1972). Functional evaluation of prolactin secretion: A guide to therapy. J. Clin. Invest. 51, 706-709.
Gautvik, K.M., Weintraub, B.D., Graeber, C.T., Maloof, F., Zuckerman, J.E., and Tashjian, A.H. Jr. (1973). Serum prolactin and TSH: Effects of nursing and pyroGlu-His-ProNH$_2$ administration in post-partum women. J. Clin. Endocrinol. Metab. 37, 135-139.
Hardy, M.H. (1950). The development *in vitro* of the mammary glands of the mouse. J. Anat. 84, 388.
Heuson, J.C., Coune, A., and Staquet, M. (1972). Clinical trial of 2-α-ergocryptine (CB-154) in advanced breast cancer. Eur. J. Cancer 8, 155-156.
Hwang, P., Friesen, H., Hardy, J., and Wilansky, D. (1971). Biosynthesis of human growth hormone and prolactin by normal pituitary glands and pituitary adenomas. J. Clin. Endocrinol. Metab. 33, 1-7.
Hwang, P., Guyda, H., and Friesen, H. (1971). A radioimmunoassay for human prolactin. Proc. Nat. Acad. Sci. USA 68, 1902-1906.
Hwang, P., Guyda, H., and Friesen, H. (1972). Purification of human prolactin. J. Biol. Chem. 247, 1955-1958.
Jacobs, L.S., Mariz, I.K., and Daughaday, W.H. (1972). A mixed heterologous radioimmunoassay for human prolactin. J. Clin. Endocrinol. Metab. 34, 484-490.
Jacobs, L.S., Snyder, P.J., Utiger, R.D., and Daughaday, W.H. (1973). Prolactin response to thyrotropin-releasing hormone in normal subjects. J. Clin. Endocrinol. Metab. 36, 1069-1073.
Jacobs, L.S., Snyder, P.J., Wilber, J.F., Utiger, R.D., and Daughaday, W.H. (1971). Increased serum prolactin after administration of synthetic thyrotropin releasing hormone (TRH) in man. J. Clin. Endocrinol. Metab. 33, 996-998.
Juergens, W.G., Stockdale, F.E., Topper, Y.J. and Elias, J.J. (1965). Hormone-dependent differentiation of mammary gland *in vitro*. Proc. Nat. Acad. Sci. USA 54, 629-634.
Kleinberg, D.L., and Frantz, A.G. (1971). Human prolactin: Measurement in plasma by *in vitro* bioassay. J. Clin. Invest. 50, 1557-1568.
Kleinberg, D.L., Noel, G.L., and Frantz, A.G. (1971). Chlorpromazine stimulation and L-dopa suppression of plasma prolactin in man. J. Clin. Endocrinol. Metab. 33, 873-876.
Kleinberg, D.L., Noel, G.L., and Frantz, A.G. (1976). Galactorrhea: A study of 235 cases. (In preparation.)
Kolodny, R.C., Jacobs, L.S., and Daughaday, W.H. (1972). Mammary stimulation causes prolactin secretion in non-lactating women. Nature 238, 284-286.
Lal, S., De La Vega, C.E., Sourkes, T.L., and Friesen, H.G. (1973).

Effect of apomorphine on growth hormone, prolactin, luteinizing hormone and follicle-stimulating hormone levels in human serum. J. Clin. Endocrinol. Metab. 37, 719-724.

Lemberger, L., Crabtree, R., Clemens, J., Dyke, R.W., and Woodburn, T. (1974). The inhibitory effect of an ergoline derivative (lergotrile, compound 83636) on prolactin secretion in man. J. Clin, Endocrinol. Metab. 39, 579-584.

Lewis, U.J., Singh, R.N.P., and Seavey, B.K. (1971). Human prolactin: Isolation and some properties. Biochem. Biophys. Res. Comm. 44, 1169-1176.

Lewis, U.J., Singh, R.N.P., Sinha, Y.N., and VanderLaan, W.P. (1971). Electrophoretic evidence for human prolactin. J. Clin. Endocrinol. Metab. 33, 153-156.

L'Hermite, M., and Robyn, C. (1972). Prolactine hypophysaire humaine: Détection radioimmunologique et taux du cours de la grossesse. Ann. Endocrinol. (Paris), 33, 357.

Loewenstein, J.E., Mariz, I.K., Peake, G.T., and Daughaday, W.H. (1971). Prolactin bioassay by induction of N-acetyllactosamine synthetase in mouse mammary gland explants. J. Clin. Endocrinol. Metab. 33, 217-224.

Malarkey, W.B. (1975). Nonpuerperal lactation and normal prolactin regulation. J. Clin. Endocrinol. Metab. 40, 198-204.

Malarkey, W.B., Jacobs, L.S., and Daughaday, W.H. (1971). Levodopa suppression of prolactin in nonpuerperal galactorrhea. New Eng. J. Med. 285, 1160-1163.

McNeilly, A.S., Evans, G.E., and Chard, T. (1973). Observations on prolactin during the menstrual cycle. In: *Human Prolactin*, pp. 231-232. Proceedings of the International Symposium on Human Prolactin, Brussels, June 12-14, 1973. Excerpta Medica, Amsterdam.

Niall, H.D., Hogan, M.L., Sauer, R., Rosenblum, I.Y., and Greenwood, F.C. (1971). Sequences of pituitary and placental lactogenic and growth hormones: Evolution from a primordial peptide by gene reduplication. Proc. Nat. Acad. Sci. USA 68, 866-869.

Nicoll, C.S., Fiorindo, R.P., McKennee, C.T., and Parsons, J.A. (1970). Assay of hypothalamic factors which regulate prolactin secretion. In: *Hypophysiotropic Hormones of the Hypothalamus: Assay and Chemistry* (Meites, J., ed.), pp. 115-144, Williams and Wilkins Co., Baltimore.

Noel, G.L., Dimond, R.C., Wartofsky, L., Earll, J.M., and Frantz, A.G. (1974). Studies of prolactin and TSH secretion by continuous infusion of small amounts of thyrotropin-releasing hormone (TRH). J. Clin. Endocrinol. Metab. 39, 6-17.

Noel, G.L., Suh, H.K., and Frantz, A.G. (1973). L-dopa suppression of TRH-stimulated prolactin release in man. J. Clin. Endocrinol. Metab. 36, 1255-1258.

Noel, G.L., Suh, H.K., and Frantz, A.G. (1974). Prolactin release during nursing and breast stimulation in postpartum and non-postpartum subjects. J. Clin. Endocrinol. Metab. 38, 413-423.

Noel, G.L., Suh, H.K., Stone, G., and Frantz, A.G. (1972). Human prolactin and growth hormone release during surgery and other conditions of stress. J. Clin. Endocrinol. Metab. 35, 840-851.

Parker, D.C., Rossman, L.G., and VanderLaan, E.F. (1973). Sleep-related, nyctohemeral and briefly episodic variation in human plasma prolactin concentrations. J. Clin. Endocrinol. Metab. 36, 1119-1124.

Posner, B.I., Kelly, P.A., Shiu, R.P.C., and Friesen, H.G. (1974). Studies of insulin, growth hormone and prolactin binding: Tissue distribution, species variation and characterization. Endocrinology 96, 521-531.

Reece, R.P., and Turner, C.W. (1937). Effect of stimulus of suckling upon galactin content of the rat pituitary. Proc. Soc. Exp. Biol. Med. 35, 621-622.

Riddle, O., Bates, R.W., and Dykshorn, S. (1933). The preparation, identification and assay of prolactin--a hormone of the anterior pituitary. Amer. J. Physiol. 105, 191-216.

Rivera, E.M., and Bern, H.A. (1961). Influence of insulin on maintenance and secretory stimulation of mouse mammary tissues by hormones in organ-culture. Endocrinology 69, 340-353.

Rogol, A.D., and Rosen, S.W. (1974). Prolactin of apparent large molecular size: The major immunoactive prolactin component in plasma of a patient with a pituitary tumor. J. Clin. Endocrinol. Metab. 38, 714-717.

Sassin, J.F., Frantz, A.G., Kapen, S., and Weitzman, E.D. (1973). The nocturnal release of human prolactin is dependent on sleep. J. Clin. Endocrinol. Metab. 37, 436-440.

Sassin, J.F., Frantz, A.G., Weitzman, E.D., and Kapen, S. (1972). Human prolactin: 24-hour pattern with increased release during sleep. Science 177, 1205-1207.

Sassin, J.F., Parker, D.C., Mace, J.W., Gotlin, R.W., Johnson, L.C., and Rossman, L.G. (1969). Human growth hormone release: Relation to slow wave sleep and sleep-waking cycles. Science 165, 513-515.

Shiu, R.P.C., Kelly, P.A., and Friesen, H.G. (1973). Radioreceptor assay for prolactin and other lactogenic hormones. Science 180, 968-971.

Sinha, Y.N., Selby, F.W., Lewis, U.J., and VanderLaan, W.P. (1973). A homologous radioimmunoassay for human prolactin. J. Clin. Endocrinol. Metab. 36, 509-516.

Snyder, P.J., Jacobs, L.S., Utiger, R.D., and Daughaday, W.H. (1973). Thyroid hormone inhibition of the prolactin response to thyrotropin-releasing hormone. J. Clin. Invest. 52, 2324-2329.

Stearns, E.L., Winter, J.S.D., and Faiman, C. (1973). Effects of coitus on gonadotropin, prolactin and sex steroid levels in man. J. Clin. Endocrinol. Metab. 37, 687-691.

Suh, H.K., and Frantz, A.G. (1974). Size heterogeneity of human prolactin in plasma and pituitary extracts. J. Clin. Endocrinol. Metab. 39, 928-935.

Takahashi, Y., Kipnis, D.M., and Daughaday, W.H. (1968). Growth hormone secretion during sleep. J. Clin, Invest. 47, 2079-2090.

Tashjian, A.H. Jr., Barowsky, N.J., and Jensen, D.K. (1971). Thyrotropin releasing hormone: Direct evidence for stimulation of prolactin production by pituitary cells in culture. Biochem. Biophys. Res. Comm. 43, 516-523.

Tolis, G., Somma, M., Van Campenhout, J., and Friesen, H. (1974). Prolactin secretion in sixty-five patients with galactorrhea. Amer. J. Obstet. Gynecol. 118, 91-101.

Topper, Y.J. (1968). Multiple hormone interactions related to the growth and differentiation of mammary gland *in vitro*. Trans. N.Y. Acad. Sci. 30, 869.

Turkington, R.W. (1971). Measurement of prolactin activity in human serum by the induction of specific milk proteins in mammary gland *in vitro*. J. Clin. Endocrinol. Metab. 33, 210-216.

Tyson, J.E., Friesen, H.G., and Anderson, M.S. (1972). Human lactational and ovarian response to endogenous prolactin release. Science 177, 897-900.

Valverde, R.C., Chieffo, V., and Reichlin, S. (1972). Prolactin-releasing factor in porcine and rat hypothalamic tissue. Endocrinology 91, 982-993.

Van Wyk, J.J., and Grumbach, M.M. (1960). Syndrome of precocious menstruation and galactorrhea in juvenile hypothyroidism: An example of hormonal overlap in pituitary feedback. Pediat. 57, 416-435.

Vekemans, M., Delvove, R., L'Hermite, M., and Robyn, C. (1972). Evolution des taux sériques de prolactine au cours du cycle menstruel. C.R. Acad. Sci. (Paris), Sér. D., 275, 2247.

Yen, S.S.C., Ehara, Y., and Siler, T.M. (1974). Augmentation of prolactin secretion by estrogen in hypogonadal women. J. Clin, Invest. 53, 652-655.

Zimmerman, E.A., Defendini, R., and Frantz, A.G. (1974). Prolactin and growth hormone in patients with pituitary adenomas: A correlative study of hormone in tumor and plasma by immunoperoxidase technique and radioimmunoassay. J. Clin. Endocrinol. Metab. 38, 577-585.

DISCUSSION AFTER DR. FRANTZ'S PAPER

Dr. Barnawell
I was particularly interested in your citing of the one instance of the mother who experienced milk letdown but no increase in prolactin. That was just one case, is that correct?

Dr. Frantz
No, there were at least two women in that category--not a large number.

Dr. Barnawell

That seems quite odd; I can imagine that letdown could occur without breast stimulation, but I should think then it would be a psychic phenomenon, which presumably would be very similar to breast stimulation.

Dr. Frantz

They are not the same. Women will sometimes get letdown without nursing and occasionally without even the conscious anticipation of nursing. In other words, it is a psychic phenomenon not necessarily mediated by tactile sensations on the breast. It is an oxytocin phenomenon, in that one can get squirting out of milk, I mean very forcible milk letdown, by injecting oxytocin into a lactating woman, as we have done. It causes myoepithelial contraction in the breast, but the prolactin doesn't go up.

Dr. Barnawell

Presumably this is hypothalamic.

Dr. Frantz

Yes, this is hypothalamic, as evidenced by the presumed release of oxytocin, but the psychic factors affecting oxytocin do not seem to be the same as those affecting prolactin.

Dr. Jacobs

I wonder if you could tell us what the open circles in the pituitary tumor category represented and give us a little information about the half dozen or so patients with pituitary tumors with apparently perfectly normal circulating levels. In my experience that is a relatively unusual occurrence. I presume these were people who were recognized radiographically to have tumors?

Dr. Frantz

No, the open circles in that slide represented patients who had undergone radiotherapy for their galactorrhea. There are only very few patients who have tumors and lactation who will have levels that are even close to the normal range. However, I think you cannot exclude a tumor if you find a level within the normal range. You still have to do skull films. But a normal prolactin is pretty good evidence against a tumor.

On the other hand, I think from a clinical point of view, it's important that prolactin levels over a certain amount rule in a pituitary tumor and in fact diagnose it. All patients with galactorrhea and with prolactins over 500 ng/ml have tumors without exception, in our experience. Most people with levels of over 200 will turn out to have tumors, and I suspect that those who don't have clinically evident sellar enlargement probably do have small adenomas which may later become manifest on radiographic examination. We have seen several patients with galactorrhea, high prolactins, and initially normal skull films who later developed frank sellar abnormalities. We also had one normal medical student in our institution, who volunteered for some studies on water loading. He had a resting prolactin of 350 ng/ml, although he was completely asymptomatic, both endocrinologically and neurologically. That, of course, led us to do a skull film and he did have an enlarged sella turcica. Incidentally, he had a normal sperm count, which rather surprised me.

Dr. Meites

I was struck by your present finding, in which contrary to some of your own earlier work and that of other people who've studied human prolactin, there is a significant difference between normal men and women in the amounts of serum prolactin present.

Dr. Frantz

Yes, that's true. There was such an overlap in our first reports that we were unable to get significant differences in the two sexes. There was a slight difference, but it was not statistically significant. Dr. Friesen initially didn't find a difference either, but later he also came to feel that there was one. So I think there is now agreement among investigators that men do have lower prolactin levels than women, though the overlap is considerable. The difference seems to come on at puberty, with a slight rise in the female levels that is presumably due to increased estrogen secretion.

Dr. Meites

I'm very happy to see that. Of course, that is parallel with the animal work that Dr. Turner reported on this morning. In practically all animal species females have more prolactin than males. As to the question about the need of prolactin for lactation in women, it has been reported, and I think you've been one of those to report this, L-dopa and ergot drugs can reduce lactation in women, suggesting that prolactin does have a role. Whether you need high levels of prolactin is another problem. It is of interest that in milk cows, by the use of ergot drugs, it has been possible to reduce serum prolactin to picogram levels without altering milk production in the slightest, suggesting that in the bovine at least, prolactin may not be extremely important for maintaining lactation. We can't say that it's of no importance, however, because there are still minute amounts present in the serum, and of course we have to keep in mind the prolactin receptors. The prolactin receptor activity is high in the mammary gland, and it's possible that the lactating bovine udder sequesters large amounts of prolactin from the circulation and holds it in the udder tissues.

Dr. Frantz

In these experiments in cows, how long has the prolactin been suppressed with ergot and how long has the lactation been maintained? Do you recall?

Dr. Meites

This has been done at our university by Dr. Allan Tucker, and it can be done for several weeks at a time. Of course the effect is almost immediate in reducing the prolactin, but it has no effect on milk production.

Dr. Frantz

In the early days of animal work, I believe that experiments were done involving the hypophysectomy of lactating animals. Wasn't that always follows immediately by cessation of milk production?

Dr. Meites

This is correct. This was first demonstrated in Dr. Turner's laboratory, and there wasn't much question about it. Of course, in the bovine this hasn't been done. In the bovine it appears that growth hormone is a very important factor for maintaining milk production, and it has been shown that administration of prolactin to the bovine has practically no effect on lactation. It was shown by Folley and his coworkers in England many years ago that growth hormone induced a very marked increase in lactation in the bovine, whereas prolactin was ineffective.

Dr. Frantz

That's interesting because bovine growth hormone doesn't have any lactogenic potency in the pigeon crop sac assay.

Dr. Meites

True, but other hormones than prolactin can influence lactation. One final thought--I wonder if you're aware of the correlation that has been reported in Boston, England, and Finland between breast cancer incidence and reserpine and related drugs. What comments do you have on that?

Dr. Frantz

That was recently reported in Lancet (Jick, Slone, Shapiro, and Heinonen, 1974; Armstrong, Stevens, and Doll, 1974; Heinonen, Shapiro, Tuominen, and Turunen, 1974). There has been at least one other study which has looked at the incidence of breast cancer in psychiatric patients treated with phenothiazines and butyrophenones, which are really better releasers of prolactin than reserpine is (Brugmans, Verbruggen, Dom, and Schuermans, 1973). This study suggested that there is not a correlation; schizophrenic patients and others maintained on these tranquilizers did not seem to have an increased incidence of breast cancer. This was a limited study and more data are needed. I think there is no question that reserpine does raise prolactin if a person takes it for a long time, and presumably there is some degree of chronic, mild hyperprolactinemia. In our hands reserpine only resulted in a doubling of prolactin levels, but that is quite a lot, of course.

In relation to the cancer studies, certainly breast cancer patients do not have higher than normal levels of prolactin in general; we have looked at a lot of them. That, of course, doesn't mean that prolactin is not playing a very important permissive role in the development of the tumor. In our own studies we have examined about 2 dozen patients with breast cancer and metastases to whom we gave L-dopa chronically. We measured the prolactin levels quite often and varied the doses of L-dopa (Frantz *et al.*, 1973). We found that we were always able to demonstrate a decrease in prolactin after each dose of L-dopa, and our studies led us to believe that we were probably reducing the 24-hour production, but we couldn't say that for sure. We didn't do any nighttime studies, and to do this well, you really have to do it with half-hour or more frequent measurements. Nevertheless, of these patients we had definite remission in two, in one of whom the remission was of six month's duration, with complete regression of widespread skin metastases. Another had a shorter duration of remission of only about six week's duration. A number of patients had relief of pain, but one cannot count that in tumor work because so many things will affect pain; L-dops itself may affect the pain threshold. We did not get radiologic healing in any patient, but we did seem to get what looked like arrest, at least of rapidly progressing bone lesions. I can't help thinking that prolactin, from your work and Dr. Pearson's work and Dr. Boot's, really has an important influence on breast cancer in some patients, and that if you could get rid of prolactin you almost surely would induce some significant remissions. I think the problem with L-dopa is that it is really not a very good chronic suppressant of prolactin; you cannot get prolactin levels down to zero and you can't keep them down. One would think that ergot would be the best drug for this purpose because ergot has a much longer duration of action and it effectively lowers prolactin levels. On the other hand, there is one published study in the European literature by Heuson (1972) which reported that in 19 patients who were given CB-154 in adequate doses, there was no incidence of remission of breast cancer at all. That is just one study, and I think much larger studies will have to be done. I think the goal, however, of trying to suppress prolactin in patients with metastatic carcinoma, particularly those who may be demonstrated to have prolactin receptors, is very worth pursuing.

Dr. Gillespie

I have a question, courtesy of one of my physician friends who is an endocrinologist at Johns Hopkins. He asked if there is any known physiologic effect of prolactin in the male.

Dr. Frantz

One that people have speculated about is a possible effect on the prostate, because animal studies have indicated that prolactin does seem to synergize with androgens in the development of accessory sex structures in the male. We have looked at this too, in patients with benign prostatic hypertrophy who came to surgery (Birkhoff, Lattimer, and Frantz, 1974). This was a very limited study, which only showed that the plasma prolactin levels bore no relation to the degree of prostatic enlargement. There is a gradual decline in prolactin in men, which extends throughout life from adolescence on, at a very slow rate, so if you take a group of elderly men they will have, on the average, perhaps only 50% or 60% as much prolactin as younger men. It is a very slow, statistically significant decline, and prostatic hypertrophy, of course, increases in the older age of men. While this does not, by any means, exclude a permissive role for prolactin perhaps in the development of prostatic hypertrophy as a disease, it certainly indicates that increased secretion does not play an initiating role. What else prolactin might be doing, I have no idea. I frankly don't think prolactin has much of a physiological role in the male.

Dr. Parsons

I have a practical question. For those of us who are doing prolactin experiments with rats and are interested in doing chronic bleeding in these animals, is there any anesthetic that we can use? Innovar, which contains the tranquilizer droperidol raises prolactin levels in rats just as in human subjects.

Dr. Frantz

I don't know. I can't answer for the rat. The rat is really a little different than the human in many respects. I think Dr. Meites would have better information on that point, because he has looked at some barbiturates in the rat. I would certainly go to a non-neuroleptic drug of some kind, but pentobarbital has been reported to have some effect on prolactin in the rat, has it not, Joe?

Dr. Meites

We reported that initially, for about a half hour, it resulted in a marked elevation of serum prolactin and thereafter in a marked suppression for a prolonged period. We haven't found any good anesthetic yet that we can use on rats that does not alter prolactin levels.

Dr. Frantz

In monkeys, we have found that phencyclidine, which is widely used as a quieting agent, doesn't seem to alter the hormonal status tremendously of these animals. I don't know what phencyclidine does in the rat or if it is any good in the rat. Baseline prolactin levels and prolactin pulsatile secretory episodes were unchanged, although there was some increase in the response to TRH.

DISCUSSION REFERENCES

Armstrong, B., Stevens, N., and Doll, R. (1974). Retrospective study of the association between use of Rauwolfia derivatives and breast cancer in English women. Lancet ii, 672-675.

Birkoff, J.D., Lattimer, J.K., and Frantz, A.G. (1974). Role of prolactin in benign prostatic hypertrophy. Urology 4, 557-559.

Brugmans, J., Verbruggen, F., Dom, J., and Schuermans, V. (1973). Prolactin, phenothiazines, admission to mental hospital, and carcinoma of the breast (letter to the editor). Lancet ii, 502-503.

Frantz, A.G., Habif, D.V., Hyman, G.A., Suh, H.K., Sassin, J.F., Zimmerman, E.A., Noel, G.L., and Kleinberg, D.L. (1973). Physiological and pharmacological factors affecting prolactin secretion, including its suppression by L-DOPA in the treatment of breast cancer. In: *Human Prolactin, Proceedings of the International Symposium on Human Prolactin*, Brussels, June 12-14, 1973, pp. 273-290 (Pasteels, J.L., and Robyn, C, eds), Excerpta Medica, Amsterdam; American Elsevier Publishing Co., Inc., New York.

Heinonen, O.P., Shapiro, S., Tuominen, L., and Turunen, M.I. (1974). Reserpine use in relation to breast cancer. Lancet ii, 675-677.

Heuson, J.C., Coune, A., and Staquet, M. (1972). Clinical trial of 2-Br-α-Ergocryptine (CB-154) in advanced breast cancer. Europ. J. Cancer 8, 155-156.

Jick, H., Slone, D., Shapiro, S., and Heinonen, O.P. (1974). Reserpine and breast cancer, report from the Boston Collaborative Drug Program, Boston University. Lancer ii, 669-671.

EVALUATION OF RESEARCH ON CONTROL OF PROLACTIN SECRETION

Joseph Meites[1]

Department of Physiology
Michigan State University
East Lansing, MI 48824

INTRODUCTION

Before the era of modern neuroendocrinology appeared on the scene about 20 years ago, when almost nothing was known about hypothalamic regulation of prolactin secretion and radioimmunoassay methods were unavailable, there already was considerable knowledge of the control of prolactin secretion, particularly in animals. Pioneer work in the laboratories of Turner, Lyons, Reece, Riddle and Bates, Foley and Cowie, in our laboratory, and others had demonstrated that estrogen was a potent stimulator of prolactin from the anterior pituitary (AP), that changes occurred in pituitary prolactin content during the estrous cycle (highest on days of proestrus and estrus), that pituitary prolactin in animals was low during most of pregnancy, but increased at parturition, that thyroidectomy or thiouracil administration reduced pituitary prolactin content, and that newborn human infants had high amounts of prolactin in the urine. All of these early observations have been corroborated recently by the more sensitive and quantitative radioimmunoassays for prolactin.

Research during the past 20 years had demonstrated that the major regulation of prolactin secretion is exerted by the hypo-

---

[1]Research supported in part by NIH grants AM 94784 and CA10771.

thalamic portion of the brain. This control is very complex as at least 3 substances have been reported to be present in the hypothalamus that can inhibit prolactin release, and at least 4 substances that can increase prolactin release. (<u>Release</u> is used here synonymously with <u>secretion</u> since most or all of the hypothalamic agents that alter prolactin release also alter synthesis.) In addition to hypothalamic regulation, some hormones and drugs can act directly on the AP to increase or decrease prolactin release. Despite the complexity in regulation of prolactin release by so many agents, probably more in known today about how to depress or elevate prolactin release than about any other AP hormone. An attempt will be made here to evaluate critically the work on each of the major agents involved in control of prolactin secretion, particularly in light of some of the more recent findings relevant to this problem.

Prolactin Release Inhibiting Factor (PIF) of the Hypothalamus

Early work by Desclin (1950) and Everett (1954) suggested that prolactin secretion was chronically inhibited by the central nervous system (CNS). When they removed the AP from its *in situ* site and transplanted it underneath the kidney capsule in female rats, they observed that prolactin secretion apparently continued at basal or greater than basal levels, as indicated by persistence of active corpora lutea or development of the mammary gland. Secretion of all other AP hormones was depressed as indicated by atrophy of the thyroid and adrenal cortex, failure of follicular growth and ovulation, and depression of general body growth. Other evidence also indicated that the CNS chronically inhibited prolactin release, i.e., when lesions were placed in the basal tuberal region of the hypothalamus, lactation was initiated in rabbits and cats and pseudopregnancy was induced in rats; stalk transection also resulted in lactation; cultures of AP continued to synthesize and release prolactin for prolonged periods (Meities, Nicoll, and Talwalker, 1963).

The above observations led to attempts by our laboratory (Meites *et al.*, 1963; Meites and Clemens, 1972; Meities, Lu, Wuttke, Welsch, Nagasawa, and Quadri, 1972) and by Pasteels (1961) to make extracts of the hypothalamus to see whether they could inhibit prolactin secretion. Our first report (Meities, Talwalker, and Nicoll, 1960) showed that when such extracts were injected into estrogen-primed rats, they actually could initiate mammary secretion and we concluded that the hypothalamus probably contains a prolactin releasing factor (PRF). Using essentially the same procedure, Mishkinsky, Khazen, and Sulman (1968) also initiated lactation with hypothalamic extracts in estrogen-primed rats, and also concluded that this constituted evidence for the presence of PRF. However, with neutralized acid extracts of hypothalamus were tested *in vitro*, they were found to depress prolactin release and synthesis (Talwalker, Ratner, and Meites, 1963). We named the presumed hypothalamic inhibitor of prolactin secretion, "prolactin inhibiting factor" (PIF). A semiquantitative *in vitro* bioassay method was developed for measuring hypothalamic PIF activity, and it was demonstrated that many procedures could alter PIF activity. Thus suckling or administration of estrogen or tranquiliziang drugs such as reserpine, reduced hypothalamic PIF activity and increased prolactin release, whereas administration of high doses of prolactin, ergot drugs, L-dopa, or iproniazid elevated hypothalamic PIF activity and decreased prolactin release (Meites *et al.*, 1963; Meites and Clemens, 1972; Meites *et al.*, 1972).

What was actually being measured in all of the above experiments was total hypothalamic prolactin inhibiting activity, and we know now that in addition to the presumed PIF, catecholamines and acetylcholine are present in the hypothalamus, and these also can inhibit prolactin release. Furthermore, the presence of at least four substances in the hypothalamus [PRF, serotonin, thyrotropin releasing hormone (TRH), and prostaglandins] that can elevate prolactin release, raises the possibility that a reduction in any of these substances also could result in a fall in prolactin release. Thus prolactin release at any particular time reflects the sum total of all the inhibiting and stimulating influences being exerted on the AP. Despite these problems, there is some evidence that a separate PIF entity that is neither catecholamine nor acetylcholine exists in the hypothalamus (Takahara, Arimura, and Schally, 1974).

Prolactin Releasing Factor (PRF) of the Hypothalamus

Mention already has been made of early evidence that hypothalamic extracts could initiate mammary secretion in estrogen-primed female rats (Meites *et al.*, 1960; Mishkinsky *et al.*, 1968). Additional evidence was the observation that hypothalamic extracts made from six different avian species (pigeon, chicken, quail, turkey, duck, and tri-colored blackbird) showed only prolactin releasing activity. Indeed, the pituitary of these species apparently releases little or no prolactin in the absence of hypothalamic stimulation. Other evidence was that rat hypothalamic extracts could exhibit sequential PIF and PRF activities during *in vitro* incubation with rat AP tissue (Nicoll, Fiorindo, McKennee, and Parsons, 1970), that PIF and PRF activities were present in different parts of the hypothalamus (Krulich, Quijada, and Illner, 1971) and that PRF could be chromatographically separated from other hypothalamic factors (Valverde, Chieffo, and Reichlin, 1972). Some of the most convincing evidence from our laboratory was the observation that administration of drugs such as chlorpromazine could overcome prolactin inhibition by ergot drugs (Lu and Meites, unpublished), and that electrochemical stimulation of the hypothalamus could counteract sodium pentobarbital inhibition of prolactin release (Wuttke, Galato, and Meites, 1972). Both ergot drugs and sodium pentobarbital can act <u>directly</u> on the AP to inhibit prolactin release, and hence it appeared logical that a stimulating agent must come from the hypothalamus to overcome this inhibition.

The same problems apply to establishing the definite existence of a distinctive PRF in the hypothalamus as for PIF. The other substances in the hypothalamus that can increase prolactin release --serotonin, TRH, and prostaglandins--may account for all of the PRF activity of the hypothalamus. As with PIF, until a definite PRF molecule has been isolated, its existence cannot be considered as definite.

Catecholamines (CAs)

Early work by several investigators suggested that adrenergic and cholinergic drugs may have a role in release of AP hormones. Both CAs and acetylcholine are present in the hypothalamus. Sawyer, Markee, and Townsend (1949) reported that both adrenergic and cholinergic drugs could induce ovulation in rats or rabbits, and that anti-adrenergic or anti-cholinergic drugs could inhibit ovulation. Subsequently it was confirmed that catecholamines could promote LH and FSH release but inhibited prolactin release (McCann, Dhariwal, and Porter, 1968; Meites *et al.*, 1963; Meites and Clemens, 1972; Meites *et al.*, 1972). The first indication that CAs could inhibit prolactin release was a report from our laboratory (Mizuno, Talwalker, and Meites, 1964) that iproniazid, a monoamine oxidase inhibitor that prevents catabolism of CAs and therefore elevates CA activity, inhibited postpartum lactation. Subsequently it was demonstrated that administration of iproniazid and other monoamine inhibitors, as well as administration of L-dopa--the precursor of the CAs--could inhibit release of prolactin (Meites *et al.*, 1973; Meites and Clemens, 1972; Meites *et al.*, 1972). On the other hand, administration of agents that reduced synthesis or otherwise depressed CA activity, such as α-methyl-para tyrosine, reserpine, chlorpromazine, haloperidol or methyldopa, all produced a rapid elevation of prolactin release. This and the study of related changes in hypothalamic CA activity by stimuli that altered release of prolactin (Meites *et al.*, 1963), provided strong support for a role by CAs in regulating prolactin release.

There are several important questions in connection with the role of CAs in prolactin release. One is that CAs can act <u>directly</u> on the AP *in vitro* in very small doses to inhibit the release of prolactin (Meites and Clemens, 1972; Meites *et al.*, 1972), raising the question as to whether hypothalamic mediation is required for this CA action. The other, arising partly from the first, is the view that the CAs in the hypothalamus actually account for all the prolactin release inhibiting activity of the hypothalamus and actually may be the presumed PIF (MacLeod andLehmeyer, 1972). Evidence that CAs act via the hypothalamus is that injection of dopamine in the portal blood (Kamberi, Mical, and Porter, 1971a), and that systemic administration of L-dopa to rats increases PIF activity both in the hypothalamus and systemic circulation (Meites, et al., 1963; Meites and Clemens, 1972; Meites et al., 1972). However, the possibility cannot be excluded that the PIF activity measured in the hypothalamus and blood actually consisted of CAs. In favor of the view that CAs account for all the PIF activity of the hypothalamus is the recent report (Shaar and Clemens, 1974) that extraction of CAs from the hypothalamus of rats eliminated all PIF activity. However, other workers have reported the presence of hypothalamic PIF that presumably is free of CAs (Schally, Arimura, Takahara, Redding, and Dupont, 1974). Therefore, the question remains open as to the identity of hypothalamic PIF

Recently we found that CAs may be involved in the suckling-induced release of prolactin in the rat (Chen, Mueller, and Meites, unpublished). Litters of 4-day postpartum rats were removed for 8 hours and then replaced to permit suckling for 30 minutes, followed by removal of blood samples for radioimmunoassay of prolactin and growth hormone (GH). It can be seen (Figure 1) that suckling resulted in a significant elevation in both GH and prolactin. Injection of 12 mg L-dopa into mother rats just prior to returning them to their litters completely prevented the suckling-induced rise in serum prolactin, and raised serum GH to higher levels than when not given L-dopa. Injection of 80 μg somatostatin just prior to replacement of mothers with their litters prevented the rise in serum GH, but had no effect on the increase in serum prolactin (Figure 2). Suckling in postpartum lactating rats results in reduced hypothalamic PIF activity (Meites et al., 1963), and may be associated with a decrease in hypothalamic dopaminergic activity (Fuxe and Hökfelt, 1969). L-dopa administration just prior to suckling apparently prevents any fall in hypothalamic CA activity. These observations also indicate that somatostatin does not influence prolactin release.

Cholinergic Drugs. Relatively little work has been reported on the relation of cholinergic drugs to prolactin release. Libertun and McCann (1973) noted that intraventricular injection of relatively huge doses of atropine, a cholinergic blocking drug, inhibited the release of prolactin, LH and FSH in the rat. This suggested that acetylcholine stimulates release of all three hormones. However, a recent report from our laboratory (Grandison, Gelato, and Meites, 1974) indicated that cholinergic drugs inhibit prolactin release. Injection of acetylcholine into the lateral ventricles or systemic injection of pilocarpine or physostigmine, two cholinergic drugs, all decreased serum prolactin values in rats. Other

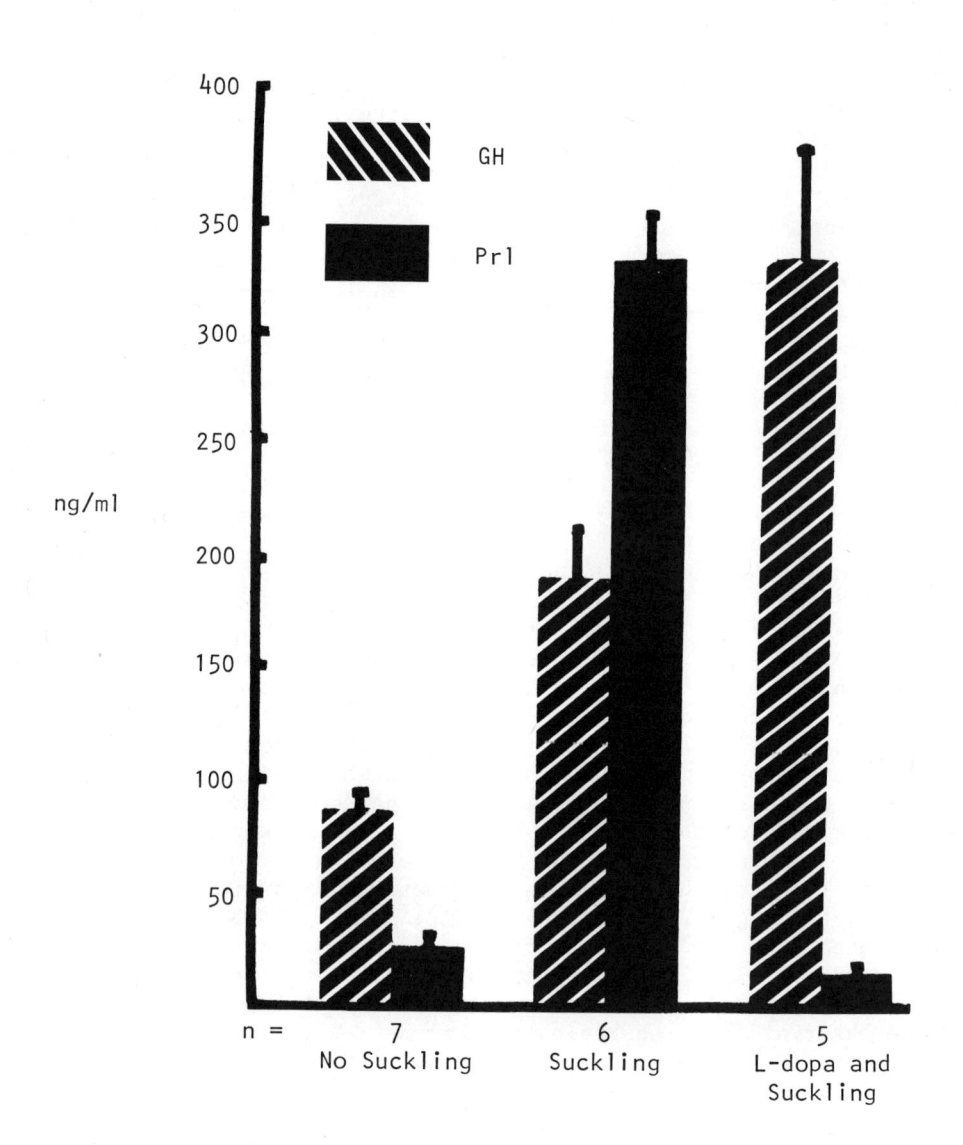

Figure 1. Effects of suckling for 30 minutes and of injection of L-dopa (12 mg/rat) just prior to suckling on serum GH and prolactin concentration in mother rats. Litters were adjusted to 8 pups each, and were removed from mothers for 8 hours prior to resuming suckling. Note that L-dopa completely prevented the suckling-induced rise in serum prolactin, but produced a greater elevation in serum GH. Numbers underneath bars indicate number of mother rats per treatment.

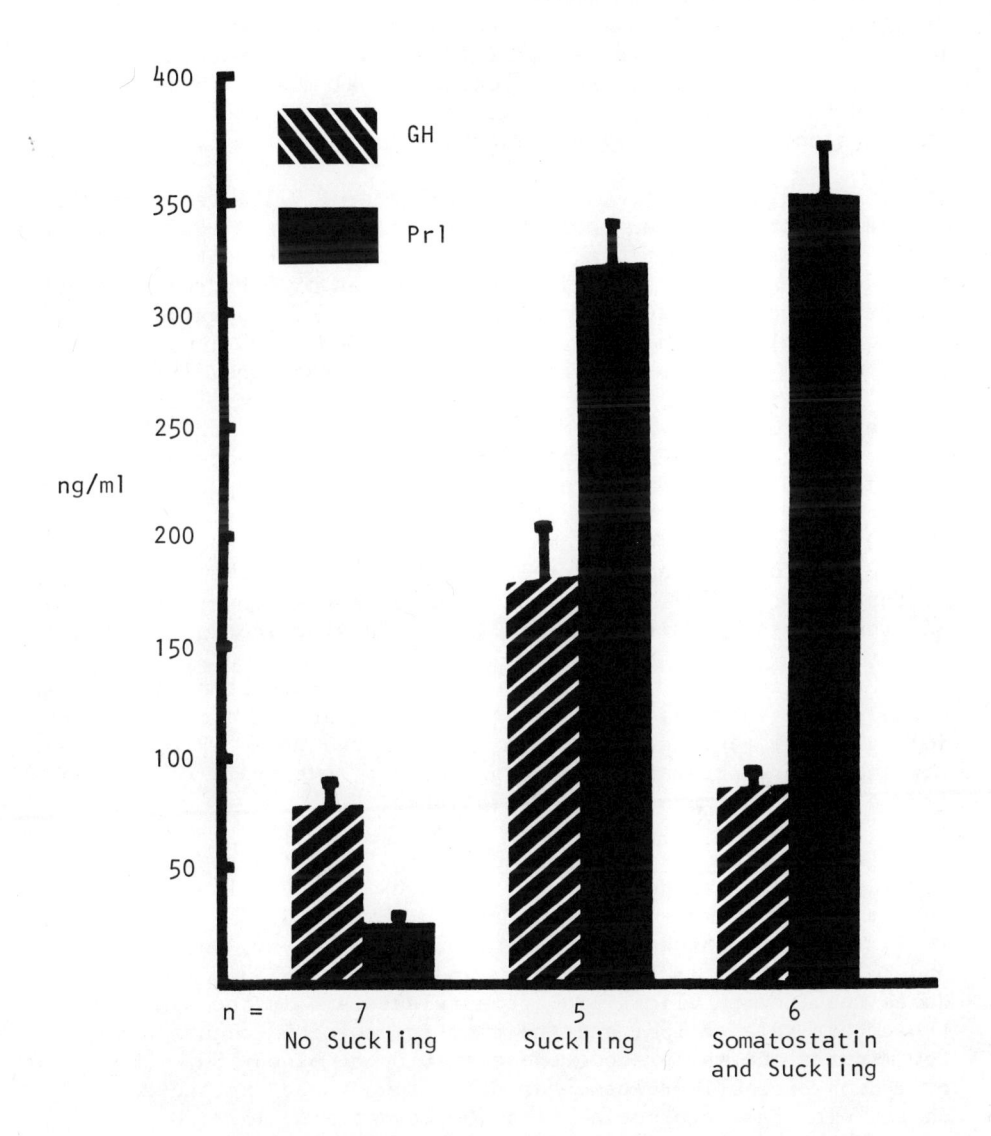

Figure 2. Effects of suckling for 30 minutes and of injection of synthetic somatostatin (40 μg/rat) once just prior to suckling and again 15 minutes later on serum GH and prolactin concentration in mother rats. Note that somatostatin completely prevented the rise in serum GH, but had no effect on serum prolactin. Numbers underneath bars indicate number of mother rats per treatment.

work (Grandison *et al.*, unpublished) suggests that the action of the cholinergic drugs is mediated through the CAs. There is no evidence that acetylcholine exerts any direct action on pituitary prolactin release (Meites *et al.*, 1963), and it can be assumed that its action is mediated via the hypothalamus. A definite role for hypothalamic acetylcholine in the control of prolactin secretion has not been established as yet.

Serotonin. Kamberi, Mical, and Porter (1971b) reported that a single injection of serotonin or melatonin into the third ventricle could increase serum prolactin in the rat. Subsequently it was reported that systemic injection of tryptophan or 5-hydroxytryptophan, the precursors of serotonin and melatonin, produced rapid elevation of blood prolactin in rats (Meites and Clemens, 1972; Meites *et al.*, 1972) and in human subjects (Turkington and MacIndoe, 1974). Apparently these indoleamines do not decrease hypothalamic PIF activity (Meites and Clemens, 1972: Meites *et al.*, 1972) and therefore may act by increasing PRF activity. Serotonin can elevate both TSH and prolactin in the serum of rats (Chen and Meites, unpublished), and the possibility exists that it may stimulate hypothalamic release of TRH. There is no evidence that serotonin can act directly on the AP to promote prolactin release (Meites and Clemens, 1972; Meites *et al.*, 1972). These and related observations suggest that serotonin acts oppositely to CAs to regulate prolactin release.

Prostaglandins. Several prostaglandins have been reported to evoke prolactin release under both *in vitro* and *in vivo* conditions (Ojeda, Harms, and McCann, 1974; Vermouth and Deis, 1972). Prostaglandins are present in the hypothalamus, but their role in prolactin release remains to be established.

Thyrotropin Releasing Hormone (TRH). TRH (pyro-glutamyl-histidyl-proline amide) not only releases TSH but also prolactin in humans and animals (Bowers, Friesen, Hwang, Guyda, and Folkers, 1971; Tashjian, Barowsky, and Jensen, 1971; Convey, Tucker, Smith, and Zolman, 1973; Mueller, Chen, and Meites, 1973). The small doses required to elicit prolactin release are in the same range as those that release TSH, and the rise in prolactin occurs within a few minutes and may precede the elevation of blood TSH. The action of TRH on prolactin release has been shown to be exerted directly on the pituitary prolactin cells (Convey *et al.*, 1973; Mueller *et al.*, 1973). These and related observations have raised the question of whether TRH is a physiological releasor of prolactin. Most of the evidence suggests that it is not, since conditions that result in release of prolactin usually do not result in a concomitant release of TSH or may even produce a decrease in TSH release.

Recently we have studied the effects of temperature on release of TSH and prolactin in male rats. Control rats were maintained at a temperature of 24°C and experimental rats at a temperature of 40°C

Table 1. EFFECTS OF HEAT AND COLD ON BLOOD LEVELS OF TSH AND PROLACTIN IN MALE RATS

Treatment and No. of Rats	Serum TSH µg/ml	Serum PRL µg/ml
Controls, 24°C (8)	.46 ± .08*	25 ± 3
Heat, 40°C for 30 min. (8)	.12 ± .02[b]	123 ± 8[b]
Cold, 4°C for 2 hr. (7)	.84 ± .16[a]	6 ± 1[b]

*Mean ± standard error of mean
[a] $p < .05$; [b] $p < .001$
(from Mueller, Chen, Dibbet, Chen, and Meites, unpublished)

for 30 minutes or 4°C for two hours. Blood samples were withdrawn immediately after removing the rats from the warm or cold temperature and these were assayed for serum TSH and prolactin by standard radioimmunoassay procedures. The results are shown in Table 1. It can be seen that heat significantly decreased serum TSH concentration, whereas cold significantly increased serum TSH values. On the other hand, heat resulted in a marked rise in serum prolactin and cold produced a significant fall in serum prolactin. Wetteman and Tucker (1974) observed similar effects of warm and cold temperatures on serum prolactin levels in cattle. The results observed here on serum TSH are in accord with many previous reports on the effects of temperature on release of TSH and thyroid hormones, but it is obvious that the effects of temperature changes on prolactin were just the opposite to those in TSH. Reichlin and Mitnick (1973) have reported that cold temperature produces an increase in hypothalamic TRH release, but if so, it is clear that this does not result in a rise in prolactin release. The mechanisms responsible for the temperature-induced changes in prolactin release remain to be explored.

Other evidence that prolactin and TSH release are controlled by different mechanisms is based on studies of the actions of central acting drugs. We recently determined the effects of a single intraperitoneal (ip) or intravenous (iv) injection of the following drugs on serum prolactin and TSH: 5-hydroxytryptophas (5HPT), the precursor of serotonin; para-chloro-amphetamine (PCA), which inhibits serotonin activity; L-dopa, which increases CAs; pilocarpine, which simulates acetylcholine action. Table 2 shows that 5HTP produced an elevation in both serum prolactin and TSH, whereas PCA administration caused a fall in both prolactin and TSH. The present results indicate that serotonin stimulates release of TSH as well as of prolactin, but this does not mean that this action necessarily is mediated via release of TRH. L-dopa and pilocarpine each produced a marked fall in serum prolactin, in agreement with pre-

Table 2. EFFECTS OF A SINGLE INJECTION OF DRUGS ON SERUM PROLACTIN (PRL) AND TSH IN ESTROGEN-PRIMED OVARIECTOMIZED RATS

Treatment and No. of Rats		Serum PRL and TSH (ng/ml)	
		Pretreatment	Posttreatment
Controls (7)	PRL	174 + 28*	158 + 23
(0.5 ml 8.7% NaCl, ip)	TSH	346 + 35	298 + 19
5HTP (12)	PRL	156 + 21	569 + 54[c]
(30 mg/rat, ip)	TSH	302 + 32	750 + 53[c]
PCA (7)	PRL	174 + 11	54 + 9[b]
(3 mg/rat, ip)	TSH	317 + 41	137 + 17[a]
L-dopa (7)	PRL	203 + 23	18 + 4[c]
(30 μg/rat, iv)	TSH	279 + 43	221 + 35
Pilocarpine (7)	PRL	181 + 14	33 + 3[b]
(10 μg/kg, ip)	TSH	286 + 32	260 + 29

*Mean ± standard error of mean
[a] $p < .05$; [b] $p < .01$; [c] $p < .001$
(from Chen and Meites, unpublished)

vious observations, but had no significant effect on serum TSH (see Table 3). This indicates that neither adrenergic nor cholinergic stimulation alters TSH release. L-dopa also had been reported not to significantly alter or to slightly reduce blood TSH levels in man (Rapoport, Refetoff, Fand, and Friesen, 1973).

Other evidence that release of prolactin and TSH are controlled mainly by different mechanisms is that stresses in general result in increased release of prolactin (Meites and Clemens, 1972; Meites et al., 1972) but in decreased TSH-thyroid hormone release (Reichlin, 1966), and that low or high doses of estrogen promote prolactin release (Meites et al., 1963; Meites and Clemens, 1972) but high doses of estrogen inhibit TSH release (Dibbet, Bruni, Mueller, Chen, and Meites, 1973). Also in postpartum lactating women, suckling produces rapid elevation of serum prolactin but has no effect on serum TSH (Bowers, personal communication).

Other Agents that Influence Prolactin Release. Some hormones and drugs can act directly on the AP to alter prolactin release, and several of these act both directly and via the hypothalamus. There is convincing evidence that estrogen, an important promotor of prolactin release in animals and in man, can directly stimulate the pituitary to increase synthesis and release of prolactin under both in vitro and in vivo conditions (Meites et al., 1963; Meites

Table 3. EFFECTS OF TRH ON PROLACTIN AND TSH RELEASE IN L-DOPA-PRETREATED MALE RATS

Treatment and No. of Rats	Pretreatment	Post-L-dopa (except controls)	Post-TRH
		Serum Prolactin	
Controls (7) (vehicle)	35 ± 4*	30 ± 5	95 ± 6*
L-dopa (7) (30 mg/rat, iv)	35 ± 5	12 ± 3[a]	17 ± 5[b]
		Serum TSH	
Controls (7)	152 ± 31	181 ± 23	2871 ± 226
L-dopa (7) (30 mg/rat, iv)	184 ± 27	141 ± 18	2651 ± 207

* Mean ± standard error of mean
[a] $p<.05$; [b] $p<.01$
(from Chen and Meites, unpublished)

and Clemens, 1972; Meites et al., 1972). This was first demonstrated by culture of rat AP tissue together with small amounts of estradiol. Estrogen also acts on the hypothalamus to reduce PIF activity. Thyroxine and triiodothyronine also can directly promote prolactin release by the rat AP when cultured *in vitro* (Meites and Clemens, 1972; Meites et al., 1972). However, there is evidence that during short-term incubation, thyroxine may first decrease AP prolactin release, and this is followed subsequently by an increase in prolactin release (Dibbet et al., 1973). There are conflicting reports on the effects of hypo- and hyperthyroidism on blood levels of prolactin in animals and man. It is generally agreed that hyperthyroidism reduces the ability of TRH to raise blood prolactin levels (Jacobs and Daughaday, 1973).

The ergot drugs are powerful and apparently specific inhibitors of prolactin release. In small or moderate doses they do not alter release of other AP hormones. They have been shown by us to inhibit the growth of carcinogen-induced mammary tumors and of prolactin-secreting pituitary tumors in rats (Meites and Clemens, 1972; Meites et al., 1972). They also can inhibit lactation in rats and women. When incubated with rat AP *in vitro*, ergot drugs prevent release of prolactin. They also can inhibit release of prolactin by estrogen either under *in vivo* or *in vitro* conditions. In addition to their direct action on the AP, ergot drugs have been reported to increase hypothalamic PIF activity (Meites and Clemens, 1972; Meites et al.,

1972) and to increase hypothalamic dopaminergic activity (Hökfelt and Fuxe, 1972). Their direct action on the AP appears to be more important than their hypothalamic effect on prolactin release.

Sodium pentobarbital administration to rats results in a significant rise in serum prolactin by 30 minutes, followed by a prolonged fall (Meites and Clemens, 1972; Meites *et al.*, 1972). The initial rise in serum prolactin was reported to be associated with a decrease in hypothalamic PIF activity, but the subsequent fall apparently was mediated by a direct action of the drug on the AP. Incubation of rat AP with minute doses of sodium pentobarbital resulted in depression of prolactin release.

Insulin, vasopressin, oxytocin, and acetylcholine apparently have no direct effect on AP prolactin release. The posterior pituitary hormones also do not promote prolactin release *in vivo* (Meites *et al.*, 1963; Meites and Clemens, 1972; Meites *et al.*, 1972), contrary to views expressed earlier by Benson and Folley (1956). Testosterone and progesterone also have no direct effect on prolactin release *in vitro*, but can promote some prolactin release *in vivo*. Neither synthetic LRH nor somatostatin (GIF) appear to have any significant effect on prolactin release.

Application to Problems of Lactation and Mammary and Pituitary Tumors. Adrenal cortical hormones as well as prolactin are essential for initiation and maintenance of lactation in most species studied thus far (Meites and Clemens, 1972; Meites *et al.*, 1972). Other hormones can influence the quantity of milk produced but are not essential for lactation. Under some conditions, prolactin appears to be the major limiting factor in determining the onset or maintenance of milk secretion. Thus lactation can be initiated in animals or man by increasing prolactin secretion through administration of moderate doses of estrogen or drugs such as reserpine, chlorpromazine and haloperidol, by placing lesions in the median eminence, by sectioning the pituitary stalk, or by persistent stimulation of the nipples (Meites *et al.*, 1963; Meites and Clemens, 1972; Meites *et al.*, 1972). Established lactation can be inhibited in some animals (not ruminants) and man by administering drugs that depress prolactin secretion, such as L-dopa and ergot drugs. L-dopa and ergot drugs also have been used successfully to treat patients with inappropriate lactation (Chiari-Frommel syndrom and Forbes-Albright syndrom)(see Frantz).

Prolactin and estrogen are the two most important hormones for development and growth of mammary tumors in rats (Meites and Clemens, 1972; Meites *et al.*, 1972) and perhaps man as well. Depression of prolactin secretion by administration of L-dopa, iproniazid or ergot drugs can inhibit development in rats of mammary cancer induced by a carcinogen, 7, 12-dimethylbenz(a)anthracene (DMBA). Ergot drugs also can prevent the appearance of spontaneous mammary cancers in

C_3H female mice. It is of interest that an excess of prolactin secretion, induced by administration of drugs such as haloperidol or reserpine, or by placement of median eminence lesions, also can inhibit mammary cancer development in rats given DMBA. This is believed to be mediated through stimulation of normal mammary growth, thereby rendering the mammary epithelium refractory to DMBA. Established mammary tumors in rats, whether DMBA-induced or spontaneous, show regression upon treatment with drugs that inhibit prolactin secretion, including use of L-dopa, iproniazid or ergot drugs. Some cases of human breast cancer also have responded favorably to treatment with L-dopa or ergot drugs (see Frantz). On the other hand, treatment with drugs or direct hypothalamic manipulations that produce an increase in prolactin secretion, result in enhanced mammary tumor growth.

Experimental transplantable pituitary tumors that secrete enormous amounts of prolactin and growth hormone have been developed in rats by Dr. Jacob Furth. Administration of L-dopa or ergot drugs has been reported to rapidly depress prolactin secretion by these pituitary tumors without altering growth hormone secretion, and the ergot drugs also have reduced tumor size (Meites *et al.*, 1963; Meites and Clemens, 1972). It has been estimated that about 30% of all pituitary tumors in human subjects secrete large amounts of prolactin, and L-dopa and ergot drugs have been used successfully to reduce prolactin secretion in these patients (see Frantz).

SUMMARY

At least three substances have been reported to be present in the hypothalamus that can inhibit prolactin release, namely a PIF, catecholamines and acetylcholine. At least four substances have been reported to be present in the hypothalamus that can stimulate prolactin release, namely PRF, TRH, serotonin and prostaglandins. Neither the existence of a distinctive PIF or PRF in the hypothalamus can be considered as definitely established. The predominant action of the mammalian hypothalamus on prolactin release is inhibitory under most conditions, and is stimulatory in avian species. In addition to control by the hypothalamus, several hormones and drugs can act directly on the pituitary to alter prolactin release. The interrelationships of these agents within and without the hypothalamus on prolactin secretion are complex, and there are many questions about their mode of action. Studies on the regulation of prolactin secretion have resulted in development of many methods for either increasing or decreasing release of this important hormone, and thereby have provided opportunities for influencing lactation, growth of mammary and pituitary tumors and other tissues responsive to prolactin.

REFERENCES

Benson, G.K. and Folley, S.J. (1956). Oxytocin as stimulator for the release of prolactin from the anterior pituitary. Nature 117, 700.

Bowers, C.Y., Friesen, H.G., Hwang, P., Guyda, H.J., and Folkers, K. (1971). Prolactin and thyrotropin release in man by synthetic pyroglutamyl-histidyl-prolinamide. Biochem. Biophys. Res. Commu. 45, 1033-1041.

Convey, E.M., Tucker, H.A., Smith, V.G., and Zolman, J. (1973). Bovine prolactin, growth hormone, thyroxine and corticoid response to thyrotropin-releasing hormone. Endocrinology 92, 471-476.

Desclin, L. (1950). A propos du mécanisme d'action des oestrogènes sur le lobe antérieur de l'hypophyse chez le rat. Ann. Endocrinol. 11, 656-659.

Dibbet, J.A., Bruni, J.F., Mueller, G.P., Chen, H.J., and Meites, J. (1973). *In vitro* stimulation of prolactin secretion by synthetic TRH in rats, and influence of thyroid hormones. Program of 55th Annual Meeting of the Endocrine Society, p. A-139.

Everett, J.W. (1954). Luteotrophic function of autografts of the rat hypophysis. Endocrinology 54, 685-690.

Fuxe, K., and Hökfelt, T. (1969). Catecholamines in the hypothalamus and the pituitary gland. In: *Frontiers in Neuroendocrinology 1969* (Ganong, W.F. and Martini, L., eds.), pp. 47-96, Oxford University Press, New York.

Grandison, L., Gelato, M., and Meites, J., (1974). Inhibition of prolactin secretion by cholinergic drugs. Proc. Soc. Exp. Biol. Med. 145, 1236-1239.

Hökfelt, T. and Fuxe, K. (1972). On the morphology and the neuroendocrine role of the hypothalamic catecholamine neurons. In: *Brain-Endocrine Interaction* (Knigge, K.M., Scott, D.E., and Weindl, A., eds.), pp. 181-223, S. Karger, Basel.

Jacobs, L.S. and Daughaday, W.H. (1974). Pathophysiology and control of prolactin secretion in patients with pituitary and hypothalamic disease. In: *Human Prolactin* (Pasteels, J.L. and Robyn, C., eds.), pp. 189-205, Excerpta Medica, Amsterdam.

Kamberi, I.A., Mical, R.S., and Porter, J.C. (1971a). Effect of anterior pituitary perfusion and intraventricular injection of catecholamines on prolactin release. Endocrinology 88, 1012-1020.

Kamberi, I.A., Mical, R.S., and Porter, J.C. (1971b). Effects of melatonin and serotonin on the release of FSH and prolactin. Endocrinology 88, 1288-1293.

Krulich, L., Quijada, M., and Illner, P. (1971). Localication of prolactin-inhibiting factor, prolactin-releasing factor (PRF), growth hormone-RF (GRF) and GIF activities in the hypothalamus of the rat. Program of 53rd Annual Meeting of The Endocrine Society, San Francisco, p. A-83.

Libertun, C. and McCann, S.M. (1973). Blockade of the release of gonadotropins and prolactin by subcutaneous or intraventricular injection of atropine in male and female rats. Endocrinology 92, 1714-1724.

MacLeod, R.M. and Lehmeyer, J.E. (1972). Regulation of the synthesis and release of prolactin. In: *Lactogenic Hormones* (Wolstenholme, G.E.W. and Knight, J., eds.), pp. 53-76, Churchill Livingstone, London.

McCann, S.M., Dhariwal, A.P.S., and Porter, J.C. (1968). Regulation of the adenohypophysis. Ann. Rev. Physiol. 30, 589-640.

Meites, J. and Clemens, J.A. (1972). Hypothalamic control of prolactin secretion. Vitamins and Hormones 30, 162-221.

Meites, J., Lu, K.H., Wuttke, W., Welsch, C.W., Nagasawa, H., and Quadri, S.K. (1972). Recent studies on functions and control of prolactin secretion in rats. Recent Prog. Hormone Res. 28, 741-526.

Meites, J., Nicoll, C.S., and Talwalker, P.K. (1963). The central nervous system and the secretion and release of prolactin. In: *Advances in Neuroendocrinology* (Nalbandov, A.V., ed.), pp. 238-288, University of Illinois Press, Urbana, IL.

Meites, J., Talwalker, P.K., and Nicoll, C.S. (1960). Initiation of lactation in rats with hypothalamic or cerebral tissue. Proc. Soc. Exp. Biol. Med. 103, 298-300.

Mishkinsky, J., Khazen, K., and Sulman, F.G. (1968). Prolactin-releasing activity of the hypothalamus in post-partum rats. Endocrinology 82, 611-613.

Mizuno, H., Talwalker, P.K., and Meites, J. (1964). Inhibition of mammary secretion in rats by iproniazid. Proc. Soc. Exp. Biol. Med. 115, 604-607.

Mueller, G.P., Chen, H.J., and Meites, J. (1973). *In vivo* stimulation of prolactin release in the rat by synthetic TRH. Proc. Soc. Exp. Biol. Med. 144, 613-615.

Nicoll, C.S., Fiorindo, R.P., McKennee, C.T., and Parsons, J.A. (1970). Assay of hypothalamic factors which regulate prolactin secretion. In: *Hypophysiotropic Hormones of the Hypothalamus: Assay and Chemistry* (Meites, J., ed.), pp. 115-144, The Williams and Wilkins Co., Baltimore.

Ojeda, S.R., Harms, P.G., and McCann, S.M. (1974). Central effect of Prostaglandin, E_1 (PGE_1) on prolactin release. Endocrinology 95, 613-618.

Pasteels, J.L. (1961). Secretion de prolactine par l'hypophyse en culture de tissues. C.R. Acad. Sci. 253, 2140-2142.

Rapoport, B., Refetoff, S., Fang, V.S., and Friesen, H.G. (1973). Suppression of serum thyrotropin (TSH) by L-Dopa in chronic hypothyroidism: Interrelationships in the regulation of TSH and prolactin secretion. J. Clin. Endocrinol. Metab. 36, 256-262.

Reichlin, S. (1966). Congrol of thyrotropic hormone secretion. In: *Neuroendocrinology*, Vol. 1 (Martini, L. and Ganong, W.F., eds.), pp. 445-536, Academic Press.

Reichlin, S. and Mitnick, M. (1973). Biosynthesis of hypothalamic hypophysiotrophic factors. In: *Frontiers in Neuroendocrinology 1973* (Ganong, W.F. and Martini, L., eds.), pp. 61-88, Oxford University Press, New York.

Sawyer, C.H., Markee, J.E., and Townsend, B.F. (1949). Cholinergic and adrenergic components in the neurohumoral control of the release of LH in the rabbit. Endocrinology 44, 18-37.

Schally, A.V., Arimura, A., Takahara, J., Redding, T.W., and Dupont, A. (1974). Inhibition of prolactin release *in vitro* and *in vivo* by catecholamines. Fed. Proc. 33, 237.

Sharr, C.J. and Clemens, J.A. (1974). The role of catecholamines in the release of anterior pituitary prolactin *in vitro*. Endocrinology 95, 1202-1212.

Takahara, J., Arimura, A., and Schally, A.V. (1974). Suppression of prolactin release by a purified porcine PIF preparation and catecholamines infused into a rat hypophysial portal vessel. Endocrinology 95, 462-465.

Talwalker, P.K., Ratner, A., and Meites, J. (1963). *In vitro* inhibition of pituitary prolactin synthesis and release by hypothalamic extract. Am. J. Physiol. 205, 213-218.

Tashjian, A.M., Barowsky, N.F., and Jensen, D.K. (1971). Thyrotropin releasing hormone: Direct evidence for stimulation of prolactin production by pituitary cells in culture. Biochem. Biophys. Res. Commu. 43, 516-523.

Turkington, R.W. and MacIndoe, J.H. (1974). Prolactin release-effector mechanisms in clinical disorders of prolactin secretion. In: *Lactogenic Hormones, Fetal Nutrition and Lactation* (Josimovich, J.B., Reynolds, M., and Cobo, E., eds.), pp. 413-432, John Wiley and Sons, New York.

Valverde, R., Chieffo, C.V., and Reichlin, S. (1972). Prolactin-releasing factor in porcine and rat hypothalamic tissue. Endocrinology 91, 982-993.

Vermouth, N.T. and Deis, R.P. (1972). Prolactin release induced by prostaglandin $F_2\alpha$ in pregnant rats. Nature 238, 248.

Wetteman, R.P. and Tucker, H. A. (1974). Relationship of ambient temperature to serum prolactin in heifers. Proc. Soc. Exp. Biol. Med. 146, 908-911.

Wuttke, W., Gelato, M., and Meites, J. (1972). Effects on Napentobarbital on hypothalamic PIF, LRF, and FSH-RF and on serum prolactin, LH. and FSH. In: *Brain-Endocrin Interaction* (Knigge, K.M., Scott, D.E., and Weindl, A., eds.), pp. 267-279, S. Karger, Basel.

DISCUSSION AFTER DR. MEITES' PAPER

Dr. Winnacker

Maybe I could get some information on the effect of chronic adrenergic blockade with let's say Inderal or propanolol on plasma prolactin levels. Propanolol is a very common and chronically used drug. Will it be dangerous in terms of chronic hyperprolactinemia?

CONTROL OF PROLACTIN SECRETION

Dr. Meites

We have no data on Inderal or propanolol. However, one of the problems with many drugs like L-dopa is that they are relatively short acting. Although the dosage would be important, I don't know if anyone has actually tried to chronically alter catecholamine levels over a prolonged period in humans and determined the effects on prolactin. Dr. Jacobs, could you answer that?

Dr. Jacobs

I don't believe that information is available in human subjects. There is some information on methysergide and cyproheptadine acutely in humans, with reported effects on both growth hormone and prolactin release induced by hypoglycemia and so forth, but there isn't any chronic information on either of these drugs. There is no information either acute or chronic to my knowledge that has been published on *alpha* or *beta* blockade.

Dr. Derby

I was wondering what prolactin can do to other pituitary hormones such as FSH and LH.

Dr. Meites

When we reduced prolactin secretion, this has resulted almost invariably in an elevation in FSH and LH secretion. For example, if one shuts off prolactin secretion in the postpartum lactating rat, these animals start cycling. We have inhibited prolactin secretion in prepuberal rats by injecting prolactin or by implanting a small amount of it in the median eminence (short loop feedback), and found that puberty was advanced by about a week. This is very significant when you consider that the female rat enters puberty between 35 and 40 days of age. Similarly, median eminence implants of prolactin reduce prolactin secretion during pregnancy or pseudopregnancy, resulting in termination of pregnancy or pseudopregnancy and in an increase in LH and FSH release. We don't know exactly how the mechanism works, and perhaps Dr. Farquhar can shed some light on this.

Dr. Derby

What is the long-term effect of high prolactin on the prolactin cells themselves, and is it of physiological significance? What is the effect of transplanting an additional rat pituitary on the animal's own pituitary gland? And I wonder how long-term the inhibition effect of a grafted pituitary is on the prolactin cell.

Dr. Meites

There have been some studies on the effect of pituitary transplants under the kidney capsule on the ability of the *in situ* pituitary to release prolactin, and the results are somewhat equivocal. Some studies have indicated that a pituitary transplant can chronically suppress prolactin secretion by the *in situ* pituitary. There is no doubt that transplanted pituitary tumors, which secrete enormous amounts of prolactin and GH, can markedly depress prolactin secretion by the host rat for months; in fact, the *in situ* pituitary shrinks in size. Cytologically we don't know what happens, but the secretion of both prolactin and growth hormone is markedly reduced.

Dr. Derby

Another example of a system that would be incompatible in some respects with TRH acting on both prolactin and TSH would be amphibian metamorphosis. According to the bihormonal model, that was proposed by Drs. Etkin and Gona (1967), and which I've been working on for a while, the idea that TRH would be responsible for regulating those two hormones is quite incompatible because at the time at which prolactin would be going down, at climax of metamorphosis, thyroxin levels are in fact going up. Recently we've been measuring directly, by radioimmunoassay, prolactin in the serum and pituitaries of tadpoles, froglets, and frogs. The results that I have so far, which have been submitted for publication, do seem to indicate that the bihormonal model with respect to prolactin is correct; I hope so. By measuring serum prolactin via a heterologous radioimmunoassay system, prolactin goes in the direction predicted by the model. In the tadpole, serum prolactin levels are higher; they decrease in climas animals and in the adult frog. I haven't measured thyroxin directly, but if we accept the older literature, it is going in the opposite direction.

Dr. Meites

Yes, there is the very early observation by Etkin that prolactin inhibits thyroid function and metamorphosis in tadpoles. I can't help but mention something I heard yesterday from Dr. Jacobs, suggesting the extremely novel idea that TRH may not even be physiologically involved in TSH and thyroid hormone release.

DISCUSSION REFERENCES

Etkin, W. and Gona, A.G. (1967). Antagonism between prolactin and thyroid hormone in amphibian development. J. Exp. Zool. 165, 249-258.

PROLACTIN, THE LIPOREGULATORY HORMONE[1]

Albert H. Meier

Department of Zoology
Louisiana State University
Baton Rouge, Louisiana 70803

ABSTRACT

　　Heavy stores of body fat in feral vertebrates are associated with periodic events such as overwintering and migration for which they serve as a source of metabolic energy. The timing of fattening by environmental cues suggests that neuroendocrine mechanisms are involved. The principal hormone that controls fat stores appears to be prolactin. Prolactin stimulates marked increases in fat stores in fish, amphibians, reptiles, birds, and mammals within one week of daily injections. However, the time of injection is critical. Injections given at one time of day cause increases in fat stores whereas injections given at another time of day may decrease body fat. The daily rhythm in fattening response to prolactin is entrained by the daily photoperiod but the rhythm is circadian in that it persists for at least several days in constant conditions of temperature and light. The photoperiodic entrainment appears to be mediated by the daily rhythm of blood corticosteroid concentrations. Corticosteroid injections can entrain daily rhythms of fattening responses to prolactin in all vertebrate species tested, including fish, reptiles, birds, and mammals. The phases of the daily rhythms of endogenous hormones in several species support the hypothesis that the temporal relation of the rhythms of corticosteroids and prolactin regulate the amount of body fat stores. Knowledge of the role of circadian rhythms in the neuroendocrine control of fat stores

---

[1] Assembled from studies supported by the National Science Foundation.

might be utilized to develop new and simple ways to treat leanness and obesity.

INTRODUCTION

Problems associated with human obesity have generated vast amounts of speculation as well as considerable research. The early work was largely performed by behaviorists who has been chemists. Although much as been learned regarding behavioral

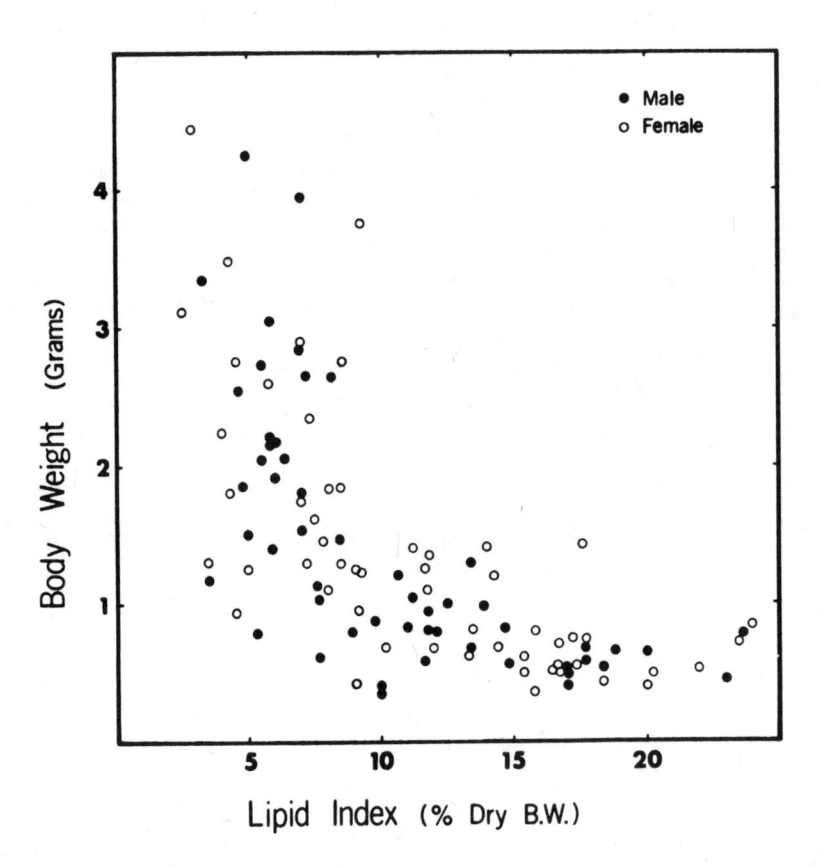

Figure 1. Lipid indexes as a function of body weight in the golden top-minnow, *Fundulus chrysotus*.

disorders, appetite centers, and lipogenic pathways, various forms of starvation in the guise of diets are still the most widely prescribed methods of reducing body weight. Many reviewers have concluded that efforts aimed at alleviating the problems of obesity have generally failed.

At this juncture it may be worthwhile to review some of the functions that fat storage has among feral vertebrates and to discuss the mechanisms that are thought to control the levels of body fat. Three principal types of fat storage that we will consider are those which are associated with development, migration, and overwintering.

FUNCTIONS OF FAT STORAGE

The level of fat stores varies during the life of many animals. In most instances younger animals have heavier stores of body fat than mature animals. Pigeon squabs, for example, have higher concentrations of body fat and are consequently more delectable than adult pigeons (Levi, 1957). The golden top-minnow, *Fundulus chrysotus*, also becomes progressively leaner as it grows and ages (Figure 1). These developmental alterations in fat stores might have a combination of ecological and physiological advantages and disadvantages. An advantage for heavy stores of body fat would be to provide a source of energy when food may be unavailable or in short supply. A disadvantage for heavy fat stores is that it imposes a greater physiological burden on the animal. The developmental alterations in fat stores suggest that the advantages may outweigh the disadvantages at certain ages.

Seasonal changes in the amounts of fat stores are often dramatic. Heavy fat stores are associated with overwintering and may be conspicuous in hibernating mammals as well as in ectothermic vertebrates that undergo a period of winter dormancy. In the green anole lizard, *Anolis carolinensis*, fat is deposited during the late summer and early autumn before the dormant period begins in November. The fat stores are gradually depleted during the winter and reach low levels in the early spring when the lizards become active and are able to secure food (Figure 2). Mammalian hibernators also accumulate heavy fat stores during an active period preceding winter and slowly utilize fat while the body temperature is reduced and locomotor activity is severely curtailed.

Perhaps the most spectacular displays of fattening are those found in migratory animals during the migratory seasons. In the white-throated sparrow, *Zonotrichia albicollis*, the total amount of body fat increases from a level of about 1.5 grams to about 5.5 grams during 7 to 10 days prior to migration. During migration the birds make frequent stops for feeding and to maintain high levels of fat stores until they reach the breeding grounds (late

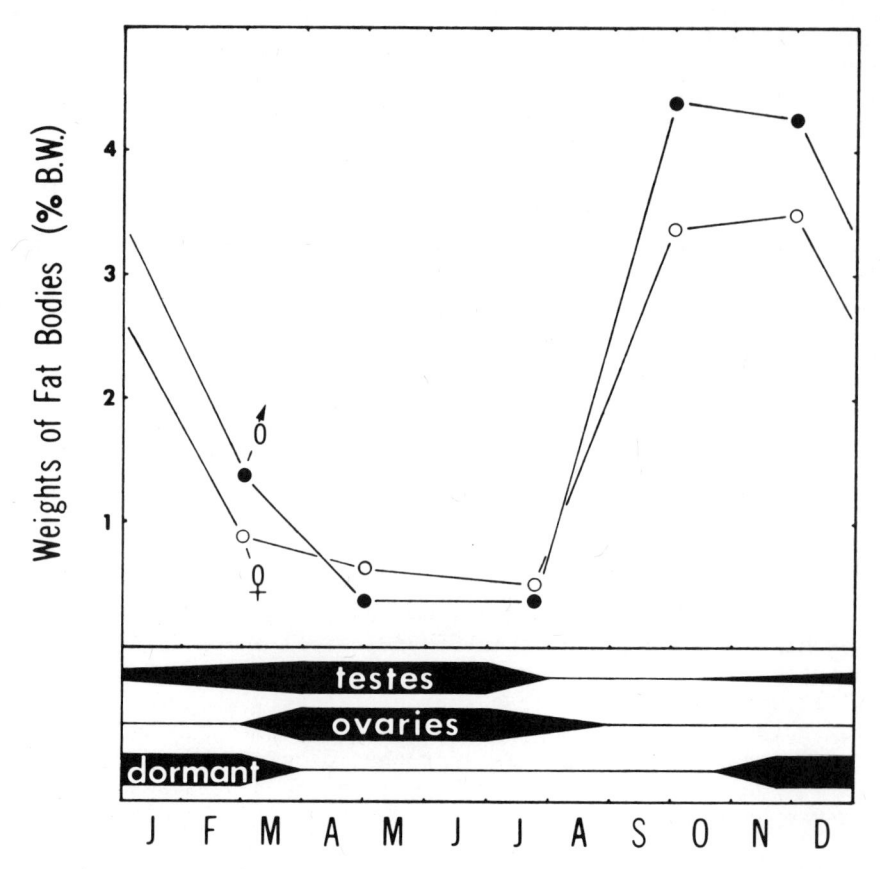

Figure 2. Annual cycle of fat body weights in the green anole, *Anolis carolinensis*. Derived from Trobec and Meier (in preparation).

spring) or the wintering quarters (late autumn)(Figure 3). The heavy fat stores during migration provide fuel for flight. The annual cycle of fat stores in the white-throated sparrow, as well as in other migrants, is associated with periods of intense locomotor activity.

The occurrence of regular seasonal fluctuations in the amounts of fat stores indicate that environmental changes during the annual cycle may influence the timing of fattening. In the white-throated sparrow, as well as in other avian migrants of the temperate zones,

the fattening that accompanies vernal migration is a consequence of
the increasing daylength of spring and can be induced during the
winter by artificially lengthening the daily photo period (review:
Meier, 1972). The annual cycle of fat stores (Figure 3), however,
is not a direct correlate of annual changes in day length. Fat
stores regress when the birds reach the breeding grounds at a time
when the daily photoperiod is at least as long as it was early in
the spring when it had a stimulatory influence on body fat stores.
In addition, fattening during the autumnal migratory period is not
initiated by changes in daylength. Thus, changes in daylength may
influence fat stores at certain times of the year, but a principal
timing mechanism for migratory fattening is within the bird itself.

Studies of fattening have been hampered by our anthropomorphic
view of fat as a societal and health problem caused by abnormal
metabolism and/or behavior. However, the periodic accumulations of

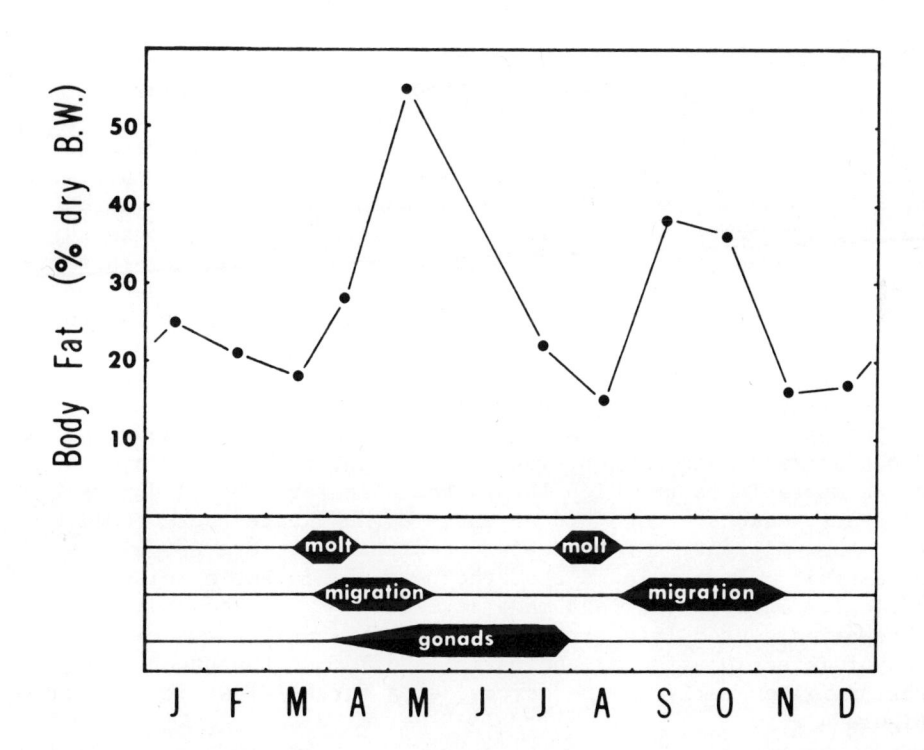

Figure 3. Annual cycle of body fat in the migratory white-throated
sparrow, *Zonotrichia albicollis*. Derived in part from
Meier, Burns, and Dussear (1969).

fat in feral vertebrates are not problems but rather solutions to problems. Thus, fat provides a source of energy for migratory flight or for overwintering. In addition, research on fattening has often been blinded by a simplistic approach wherein the amount of fat storage was considered the net effect of energy input in the form of nutrition minus the energy output of metabolism. Although this formula is undoubtedly correct as a balance equation, it seems to explain very little with respect to the control of fat stores. Increase in fat stores in migratory birds, for example, does not coincide with greatest availability of food on the one hand nor is it associated with the conservation of metabolic energy on the other.

CIRCADIAN VARIATIONS IN FATTENING RESPONSES TO PROLACTIN

Several conclusions concerning fattening among feral vertebrates are pertinent with respect to regulatory mechanisms: 1) Fattening occurs at specific times. 2) It is sometimes influenced by environmental changes. 3) It is often associated with specific events, such as migration, in which it provides a supply of energy. These conclusions suggest that the neuroendocrine system has a central role in regulating fat storage.

In searching for a possible hormonal basis for migratory fattening in birds, the mammalian literature was of little help. Most of the evidence pointed to a lipolytic effect of those hormones that might be expected to be responsive to environmental cues. On the other hand, studies of the avian endocrine system indicated that the fattening accompanying vernal migration was associated with intense endocrine activity. Despite the conflicting information, it seemed worthwhile to test the hormones of the adenohypophysis and the hormones of their target glands. Because fattening is a cumulative process, daily injections of various hormones were made over a period of a week or more. We found that one of the pituitary hormones, prolactin, could elicit enormous increases in fat stores in the white-crowned sparrow, *Zonotrichia leucophrys gambelii* (Meier and Farner, 1964). The increases in fat stores were comparable to the high levels found in feral birds during the migratory seasons. However, attempts to duplicate these results in another migrant, the white-throated sparrow, were not always successful. It developed that the time of prolactin injection was critical. Daily injections made at midday of a 16-hour daily photoperiod caused lean birds to become obviously obese within one week of injections (Meier and Davis, 1967). On the other hand, injections given early in the day caused a further loss in fat stores (Figure 4).

The presence of daily variations in fattening responses to mammalian preparations of prolactin suggested that premigratory fattening might be regulated by daily, or circadian, rhythms of

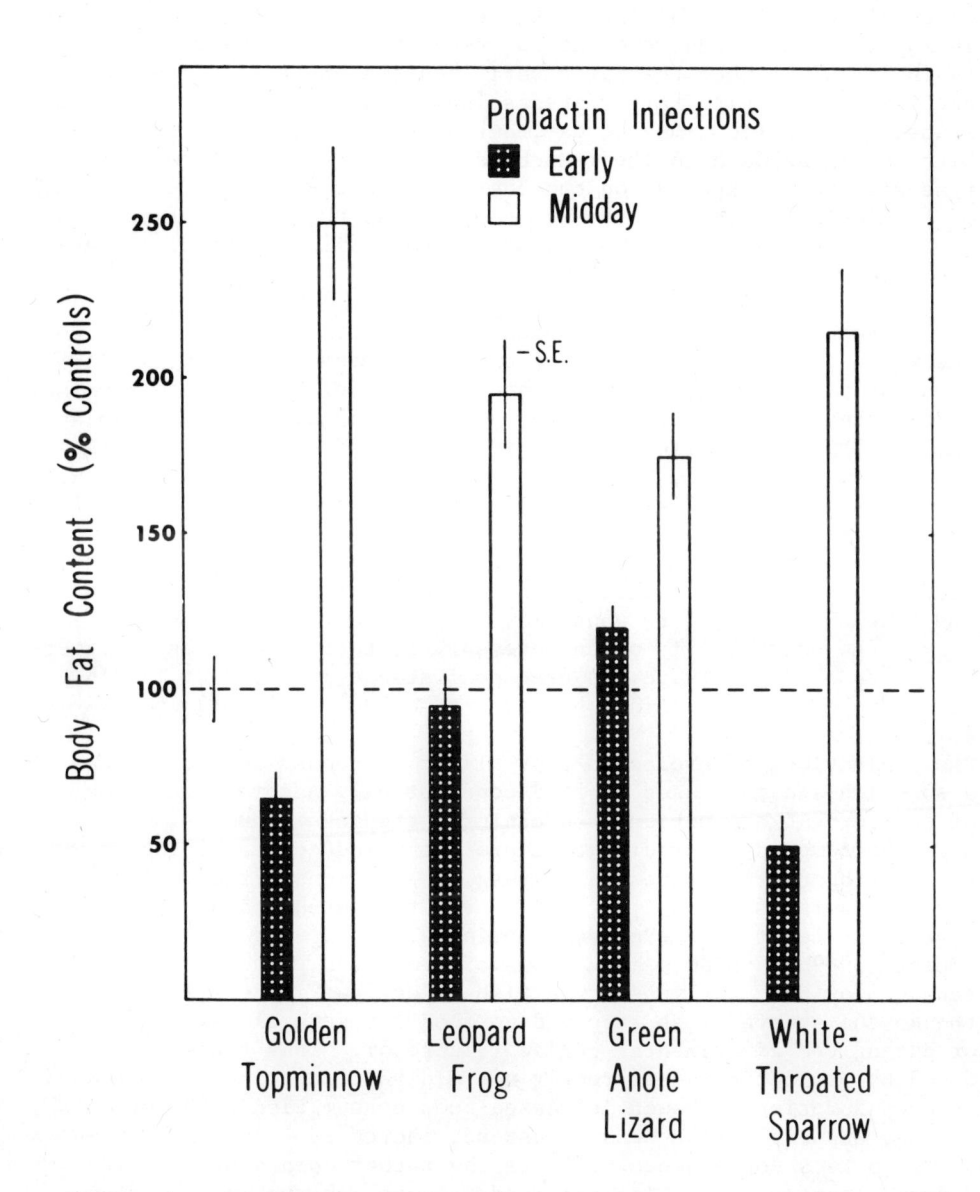

Figure 4. Variations in fattening responses to prolactin given daily for about one week either early ("dawn") or at midday (16L:8D) in several vertebrate species. Derived from Meier (1969b).

endogenous prolactin. In order to test this hypothesis pituitaries were collected from white-throated sparrows at several times of day in May when the birds were fat and ready for vernal migration and again in August when the birds were lean (Meier *et al.*, 1969). An analysis of the pituitary contents indicated that prolactin was released at specific times of day, during the afternoon in the obese birds and near dawn in the lean birds. These findings are consistent with those expected on the basis of the results of injections of prolactin and support the hypothesis that the amount of body fat stores depends in part on the phase of the daily rhythm of prolactin release from the pituitary.

Circadian fattening responses to prolactin are not limited to the white-throated sparrow. Fattening has been induced by injections of prolactin in fish (Lee and Meier, 1967; Mehrle and Fleming, 1970; Joseph and Meier, 1971; DeVlaming and Sage, 1972), amphibians (Meier, 1969b), reptiles (Meier, 1969b; Trobec, 1974a), birds (Meier and Davis, 1967; John, Meier, and Bryant, 1972), and mammals (Joseph and Meier, 1974). In all instances, the time of day when the injections are made is critical. Injections at one time of day may cause increases in fat stores whereas injections given at another time of day may cause losses of body fat (Figure 4). Because the time of fattening response may be limited to an interval of only a few hours, it is often necessary to test as many as 6 different times of day. There has been no instance in which prolactin failed to elicit fattening when such a schedule was followed.

Injections of prolactin that elicit increases in fat stores also stimulate increases in food consumption. According to some of our current assumptions concerning fattening in humans, one might be tempted to predict that prolactin induces fattening by stimulating the appetite and increasing food consumption. A test performed with starving fish has proved this assumption to be incorrect at least in the golden topminnow, *Fundulus chrysotus* (Meier, 1969b). Midday injections of prolactin produce high percentages of body fat in starved fish as well as in fed fish even though the starved fish received no food for several days before or during the experimental period (Figure 5). Thus fattening induced by prolactin is apparently not a direct reaction to increased food consumption although increased food consumption does, of course, support the process. Instead, increased food consumption seems to be a consequence of fattening rather than a primary inducer. Increased appetite and food consumption may well be reactions to changes induced by prolactin in metabolic pathways.

The manner in which prolactin influences the metabolic pathways is unclear. Although injections of prolactin *in vivo* stimulated liver enzymes involved in lipogenesis in the pigeon, *Columba livia*, the addition of prolactin to a liver culture was ineffective (Goodridge and Ball, 1967). The timing of the *in vitro* procedures

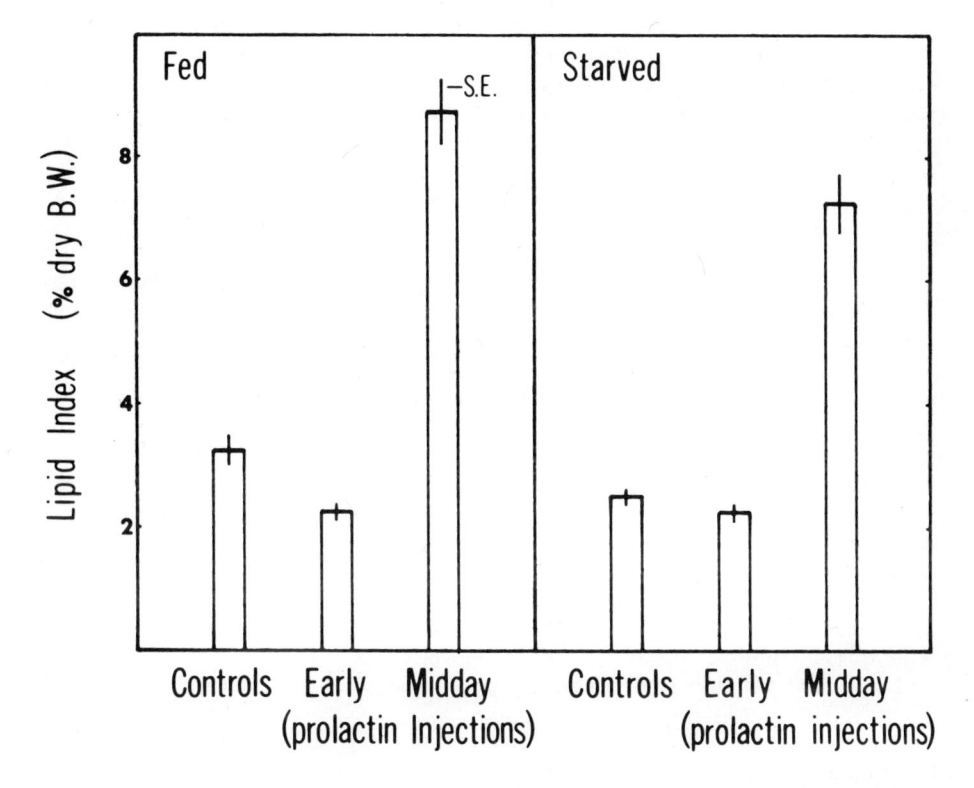

Figure 5. Variations in fattening responses to prolactin given daily for four days either early ("dawn") or at midday (16L:8D) in fed and starved golden topminnows, *Fundulus chrysotus*. Derived from Meier (1969b).

may have been inappropriate for fattening, or perhaps the removal and preparation of the culture may have altered the cellular clocks controlling the responses to prolactin. Alternatively prolactin may influence fattening indirectly.

ENTRAINMENT OF CIRCADIAN RHYTHMS OF FATTENING RESPONSES TO PROLACTIN

The presence of daily variations in fattening responses to prolactin suggests that the response rhythms are entrained by environmental cues with a 24-hour expression. In most instances involving daily rhythms, the daily photoperiod is the principal synchronizer. Entrainment of the fattening response rhythm is also effected by the daily photoperiod in the Gulf killifish, *Fundulus grandis* (Joseph and Meier, 1971). Shifting the phase of the daily photoperiod causes the appropriate shift in the fattening response rhythm. In addition, the peak of the fattening response occurs 8 hours after the onset of light whether the daily photoperiod is 8, 12, or 16 hours. Apparently the response rhythm is set by the onset of light.

The finding that the daily photoperiod entrains a daily rhythm of fattening response to prolactin suggests that the mediating system probably involved elements of the neuroendocrine system. Our principal interest was directed to the adrenal corticosteroids because of their widespread influence on metabolism and because daily rhythms of the adrenal corticosteroids have been reported in a wide range of vertebrate species. In an initial study, Gulf killifish (*Fundulus grandis*), green anoles (*Anolis carolinensis*), and common pigeons (*Columba livia*) were kept in continuous light in order to remove photoperiodic cues, and the animals were given daily injections of prolactin and corticosterone (lizards and birds) or cortisol (fish) in various temporal relations (Meier, Martin, and MacGregor, 1971). In each species there were specific times relative to the daily injection of the corticosteroids which entrained daily rhythms of fattening responses to prolactin.

A further experiment performed with Gulf killifish is of special interest. Two groups of fish were maintained on continuous light and injected with cortisol on two alternate days at either 0600 or at 1800. On the second day following the final injections of cortisol, prolactin injections were given to both groups at one of four different times of day and repeated daily for four days. Daily variations in fattening responses to prolactin were found in both groups and the phases of the two rhythms were very similar when correlated with the times of cortisol pretreatment. The persistence of the response rhythms for several days following entrainment by cortisol injections indicates that the response rhythms are circadian in a strict sense (persisting for at least two days in constant environmental conditions). It has not been determined whether the circadian response rhythm is an expression of the cells involved in fat metabolism alone or whether it also involves elements of the neuroendocrine system (Meier *et al.*, 1971).

The entrainment of daily rhythms of fattening responses to prolactin by injections of corticosteroids have now been demonstrated in species ranging from fish to mammals (Figure 6). The response rhythms are specific for each species and no general patterns are as yet discernible. The rhythms are unimodal in some species and bimodal in others. The bimodal fattening response rhythm is particularly interesting in the white-throated sparrow in that one of the hormonal patterns eliciting increases in fat stores

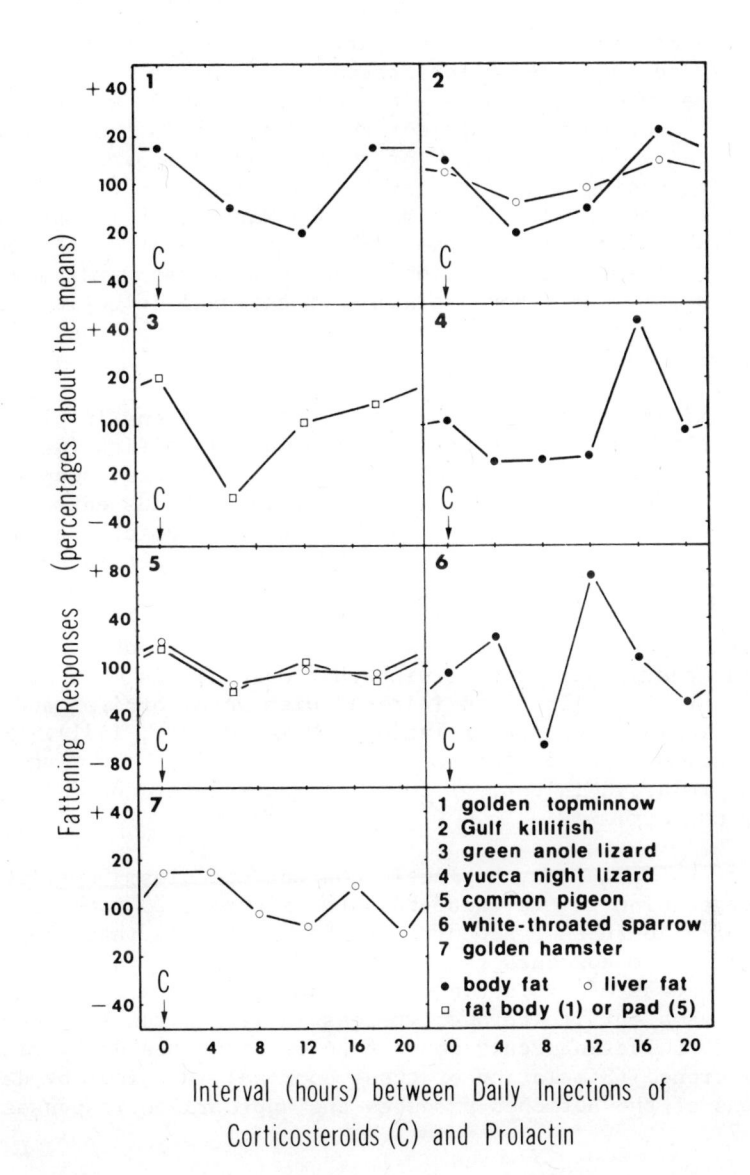

Figure 6. Daily variations in fattening responses to prolactin entrained by injections of corticosteroids in vertebrates kept in continuous light. Daily injections were made for four to ten days. All rhythms were verified statistically by analyses of variances. Derived from Meier, Trobec, Joseph, and John (1971); Meier et al. (1971); John et al. (1972); Joseph and Meier (1974); Trobec (1974a).

(injections of prolactin 12 hours after the daily injections of corticosterone) has been demonstrated to stimulate fattening and migratory behavior associated with spring migration whereas another pattern of hormones (injections of prolactin four hours after the daily injections of corticosterone) has been shown to stimulate fattening and migratory behavior associated with the fall migration (Meier et al., 1971; Meier and Martin, 1971; Martin and Meier, 1973). For example, the 12-hour relation stimulates migratory restlessness that is oriented to the north (toward the breeding grounds) and the 4-hour relation of hormonal injections stimulates migratory restlessness that is oriented to the south (toward the wintering quarters).

Determinations of corticosteroid concentrations in plasma of blood taken throughout the day from the Gulf killifish (Garcia and Meier, 1973) and the green anole (Trobec, 1974b) also support our conclusion that daily rhythms of the corticosteroids entrain the daily variations in fattening responses to prolactin. In the Gulf killifish maintained on a daily photoperiod of about 14 hours, the daily rise of plasma cortisol occurs during the afternoon, a few hours after the peak of fattening response (or about 22 hours before the daily peak of fattening response)(Joseph and Meier, 1971). This relationship agrees well with that observed in Gulf killifish kept in continuous light and injected with both cortisol and prolactin in various temporal relations (Meier et al., 1971). The greatest stimulation of fat deposition occurred in the fish that received prolactin injections 20 to 24 hours after the daily injections of cortisol.

Assays of pituitary prolactin content and plasma corticosterone concentration in the white-throated sparrow, *Zonotrichia albicollis*, provide further support for the hypothesis that the daily rhythms of these hormones regulate fat stores. In fat birds in May, the release of prolactin occurs about 12 hours after the daily rise of plasma corticosterone; whereas in lean birds in August, the release of prolactin occurs about 6 hours after the daily rise of corticosterone. Simulation of these hormonal relations by daily injections of the hormones produces the appropriate responses (Figure 7).

In the green anole kept in continuous light, the peak of fattening response to prolactin occurs when prolactin is injected at the same time as corticosterone (see Figure 6). In green anoles kept on comparable photoperiodic regimens, the daily rise of plasma corticosterone concentrations (Trobec, 1974b) and the peak of fattening responses to prolactin (Meier, 1969b) occur at the same time during the afternoon.

This collection of evidence supporting a role for the corticosteroids in mediating the photoperiodic entrainment of the daily

ROLE IN LIPOREGULATION   165

Hours after Daily Rise (R) or Injection (I) of Corticosteroid (C)

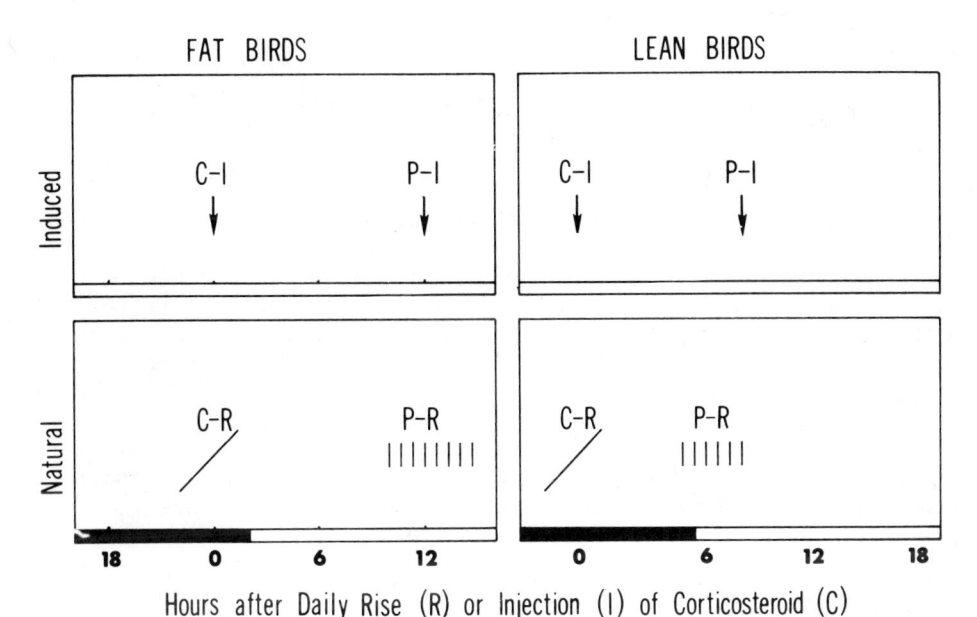

Figure 7. Daily rhythms of endogenous corticosterone and prolactin in fat and lean sparrows compared with the temporal relations of hormone injections that produce similar conditions of fat stores. Derived from Meier et al. (1969), Dusseau and Meier (1971), and Meier et al. (1971).

rhythms of fattening responses to prolactin appeared to be balanced if not entirely abrogated by the findings that the daily rhythms of fattening responses persist in hypophysectomized fish (Lee and Meier, 1967; DeVlaming and Sage, 1972). Because pituitary ACTH is necessary for the long-term maintenance of adrenal cortical function in fish as well as in mammals, it seemed unlikely that a daily rhythm of plasma corticosteroid concentration would be present in hypophysectomized Gulf killifish. Nevertheless, it is (Strivastava and Meier, 1972). Not only does the daily rhythm of plasma corticosteroid persist for at least two weeks following hypophysectomy, but the phase of the rhythm adjusts in the appropriate manner to a shift in the photoperiodic schedule. Apparently the control of the corticosteroid rhythm involves a mechanism not presently understood.

Injections of thyroxin can also entrain daily rhythms of fattening responses to prolactin in the golden topminnow, *Fundulus chrysotus* (Meier, 1970), but not in the common pigeon, *Columba livia* (John et al., 1972). In the pigeon, however, the thyroid hormones influence the phase of the circadian rhythm of fattening response and permit the retention of the rhythm that otherwise disappears after two weeks in pigeons kept in continuous light. These findings suggest that the thyroid could be involved in regulating fat stores by influencing the mechanisms controlling the responses to prolactin.

UTILIZATION OF CIRCADIAN HORMONE RHYTHMS TO REGULATE FAT STORES

Knowledge concerning roles of prolactin and corticosteroid rhythms in regulating fat stores may open up new approaches for controlling body weight and fat stores in vertebrates, including humans, For example, prolactin might be controlled so that it would be released at a specific time when it could promote either losses or gains of body fat. An obvious approach would be the use of drugs that cause a release of prolactin. Behavioral adjustments might also be expected to influence fat stores. In humans (both males and females) prolactin is released during naps (Parker, Rossman, and VanderLaan, 1973 and by stimulation of the mammary glands (Kolodny, Jacobs, and Daughaday, 1972). It might be interesting to test whether midday siestas can influence the amount of body fat stores.

The osmotic concentration of the blood has important influences on the release of prolactin in many vertebrates (Bern and Nicoll, 1969). In humans, increases in blood osmolarity stimulate the release of prolactin (Buckman and Peake, 1973). Drinking water in large amounts might be expected to decrease prolactin levels (note the relation with "water diets"). Alternatively, eating salty foods may have the opposite effects. Perhaps even the consumption of salty potato chips might be consistent with a reducing diet if it were practiced at specific times of day.

Another way to control fat stores might be to concentrate on the daily rhythm of blood corticosteroids. Under normal conditions the daily photoperiod is the principal entrainer of corticosteroid rhythms in vertebrates. However, the corticosteroid rhythm may be modified by other environmental influences and by specific behaviors provided they are repeated daily at the same time for at least a week (review: Meier, in press). In humans, an exercise program during the evening caused the establishment of a second peak of adrenal metabolites in the urine after one week. The new peak was anticipatory to the exercise program just as the normal peak is anticipatory to the onset of the daily photoperiod (or waking)(De Lacerda and Steben, 1974).

Apparently, an induction of another daily peak of endogenous corticosteroids may have accounted for the marked influence that handling has on body fat stores (Meier *et al.*, 1973). Handling disturbances repeated daily for at least 10 days can cause increases or decreases in fat stores of the golden topminnow, *Fundulus chrysotus*, green anoles, *Anolis carolinensis*, Japanese quail, *Coturnix coturnix*, and the white mouse, *Mus musculus*. Whether the disturbances cause increases or decreases in body fat depends on the time of day when the handling is performed (Figure 8). Just holding the animal for a few seconds each day is an adequate stimulus in some instances. Handling, thus, appears to produce its effect by serving as an environmental cue for entraining daily rhythms rather than as a stressor. The establishment of a new peak of corticosteroids and, consequently, of new rhythms of fattening responses to prolactin might be expected to produce new temporal relations of the hormones.

CONCLUSIONS

These findings indicate that circadian rhythms have an im-

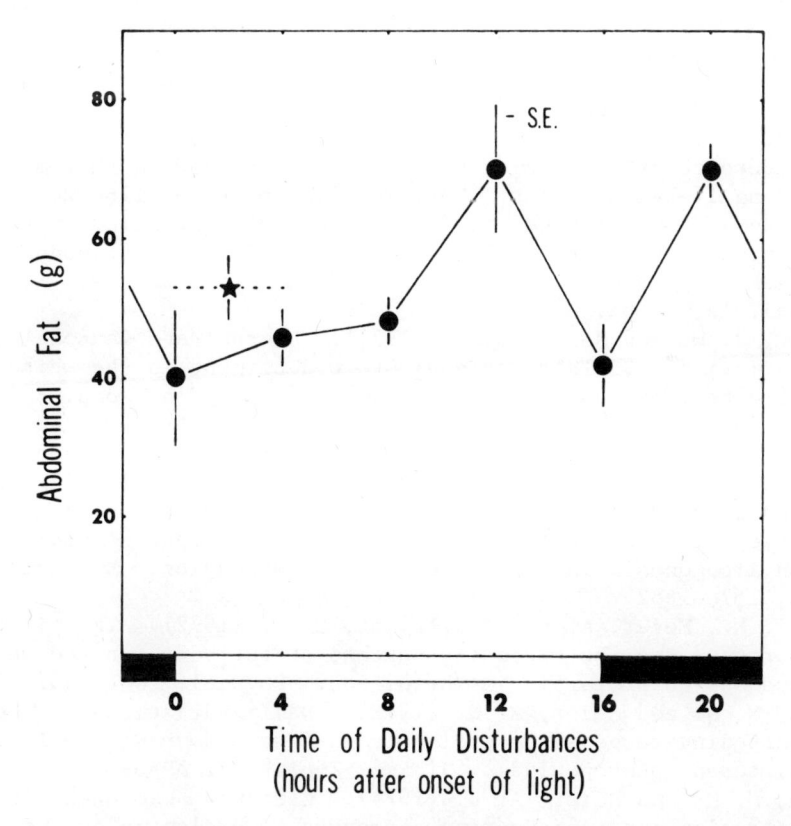

Figure 8. Daily variations in the effects of handling disturbances (saline injections daily for 10 days) on abdominal fat content in white mice. Derived from Meier *et al.* (1973).

portant organizational role in the neuroendocrine control of fat stores in vertebrates. The liporegulatory influence of prolactin should be considered one of the hormone's basic functions. With this knowledge gleaned from a comparative approach to endocrinology, we feel that new approaches in studying the control of fat stores in humans might be undertaken.

ACKNOWLEDGEMENTS

I thank my students for their contributions cited in this review, Ms. Wendie Maas for helping to assemble the review, and Ms. Christine Angelloz for typing the manuscript.

REFERENCES

Bern, H. A. and Nicoll, C. S. (1969). The taxonomic specificity of prolactins. In: *La Specificite Zoologique des Hormones Hypophysaires et de leurs activities* (Fontaine, ed.), p. 193, Centre National de la Recherche Scientifique, Paris.

Buckman, M. T. and Peake, G. T. (1973). Osmolar control of prolactin secretion in man. Science 181, 755-757.

DeLacerda, F. G. and Steben, R. E. (1974). The effect of an endurance type exercise program on the circadian rhythm of urine 17-ketosteroids. Med. Sci, in Sports 6, 126-128.

DeVlaming, V. L. and Sage, M. (1972). Diurnal variation in fattening response to prolactin treatment in two cyprinodontid fishes, *Cyprindodon variegatus* and *Fundulus similis*. Marine Sci. 16, 59-63.

Dusseau, J. W. and Meier, A. H. (1971). Diurnal and seasonal variations of plasma adrenal steroid hormone in the white-throated sparrow, *Zonotrichia albicollis*. Gen. Comp. Endocrinol. 16, 399-408.

Garcia, L. E. and Meier, A. H. (1973). Daily rhythms in concentration of plasma cortisol in male and female Gulf killifish, *Fundulus grandis*. Biol. Bull. 144, 471-479.

Goodridge, A. G. and Ball, E. G. (1967). The effect of prolactin on lipogenesis in the pigeon. *In vivo* studies. Biochemistry 6, 1676-1682.

John, T. M., Meier, A. H., and Bryant, E. E. (1972). Thyroid hormones and the circadian rhythms of fat and crop sac responses to prolactin in the pigeon. Physiol. Zool. 45, 34-42.

Joseph, M. M. and Meier, A. H. (1971). Daily variations in the fattening response to prolactin in *Fundulus grandis* held on different photoperiods. J. Exp. Zool. 178, 59-62.

Joseph, M. M. and Meier, A. H. (1974). Circadian component in the fattening and reproductive responses to prolactin in the hamster. Proc. Soc. Exp. Biol. Med. 146, 1150-1155.

Kolodny, R. C., Jacobs, L. S., and Daughaday, W. H. (1972). Mammary stimulation causes prolactin secretion in non-lactating women. Nature 238, 284-285.

Lee, R. W. and Meier, A. H. (1967). Diurnal variations of fattening response to prolactin in the golden top minnow, *Fundulus chrysotus*. J. Exptl. Zool. 166, 307-315.

Levi, W. M. (1957). *The Pigeon*, Levi Pub. Co., Inc., Sumter, S. Carolina.

Martin, D. D. and Meier, A. H. (1973). Temporal synergism of corticosterone and prolactin in regulating orientation in the migratory white-throated sparrow *(Zonotrichia albicollis)*. Condor 75, 369-374.

Mehrle, P. M. and Fleming, W. R. (1970). The effect of early and midday prolactin injection on the lipid content of *Fundulus kansae* held on a constant photoperiod. Comp. Biochem. Physiol. 36, 597-603.

Meier, A. H. (1969a). Antigonadal effects of prolactin in the white-throated sparrow, *Zonotrichia albicollis*. Gen. Comp. Endocrinol. 13, 222-225.

Meier, A. H. (1969b). Diurnal variations of metabolic responses to prolactin in lower vertebrates. Gen. Comp. Endocrinol., Suppl. 2, 55-62.

Meier, A. H. (1970). Thyroxin phases the circadian response to prolactin. Proc. Soc. Exp. Biol. Med. 133, 1113-1116.

Meier, A. H. (1972). Temporal synergism of prolactin and adrenal steroids. Gen. Comp. Endocrinol., Suppl. 3, 499-508.

Meier, A. H., Burns, J. T., and Dusseau, J. W. (1969). Seasonal variations in the diurnal rhythms of pituitary prolactin content in the white-throated sparrow, *Zonotrichia albicollis*. Gen. Comp. Endocrinol. 12, 282-289.

Meier, A. H. and Davis, K. B. (1967). Diurnal variations of the fattening response to prolactin in the white-throated sparrow, *Zonotrichia albicollis*. Gen. Comp. Endocrinol. 8, 110-114.

Meier, A. H. and Farner, D. S. (1964). A possible endocrine basis for premigratory fattening in the white-crowned sparrow, *Zonotrichia leucophrys gambelli (Nuttal)*. Gen. Comp. Endocrinol. 4, 584-595.

Meier, A. H. and Martin, D. D. (1971). Temporal synergism of corticosterone and prolactin controlling fat storage in the white-throated sparrow, *Zonotrichia albicollis*. Gen. Comp. Endocrinol. 17, 311-318.

Meier, A. H., Martin, D. D., MacGregor, R., III (1971). Temporal synergism of corticosterone and prolactin controlling gonadal growth in sparrows. Science 173, 1240-1242.

Meier, A. H., Trobec, T. N., Haymaker, H. G., MacGregor, R., and Russo, A. C. (1973). Daily variations in the effects of handling on fat storage and testicular weights in several vertebrates. J. Exptl. Zool. 184, 281-288.

Meier, A. H., Trobec, T. N., Joseph, M. M., and John, T. M. (1971). Temporal synergism and adrenal steroids in the regulation of fat stores. Proc. Soc. Exp. Biol. Med. 137, 408-415.

Parker, D. C., Rossman, L. G., and Vanderlaan, E. F. (1973). Sleep-related nyctohemeral and briefly episodic variation in human plasma prolactin concentrations. J. Clin. Endocrinol. Metab. 36, 1119-1124.

Srivastava, A. K. and Meier, A. H. (1972). Daily variation in concentration of cortisol in plasma in intact and hypophysectomized Gulf killifish. Science 177, 185-187.

Trobec, T. N. (1974a). Daily rhythms in the hormonal control of fat storage in lizards. In: *Chronobiology* (Scheving, L. E., Halberg, F., and Pauly, J. E., eds.), pp. 147-151, Igaku Shoin, Ltd., Tokyo.

Trobec, T. N. (1974b). Circadian mechanisms in the hormonal control of annual cycles of fat storage and reproduction in the lizard, *Anolis carolinensis*. Ph.D. dissertation, Louisiana State University.

DISCUSSION AFTER DR. MEIER'S PAPER

Dr. Fleming

After working with prolactin, as I have many times in hypophysectomized animals, you leave me sort of uncomfortable in the sense that maybe some of the things I've been blaming on salinities are really due to injections given a little late and injecting an hour or two later than I did the day before. I was wondering if you have any data on this kind of effect on electrolyte metabolism or things other than fat responses.

Dr. Meier

We measured plasma chloride concentrations in two teleost fishes, *Fundulus grandis* and *Fundulus chrysotus*, and found very large daily variations in the levels of this ion (Meier, et al., 1973). In addition, disturbances of handling can have a remarkable effect on the rhythm of chloride concentrations. Handling at one time of day, for example, may induce a specific daily rhythm that will persist for several days after the disturbance. In one instance the chloride concentration varied from a high of 190 mEq./liter at one time of day to a low of 95 mEq./liter. What one does to an animal prior to an experimental period may produce long lasting effects, so far as rhythms are concerned. It would be possible to obtain a wide range of results depending on when the animals are disturbed prior to the day of sampling as well as the time of day when the samples are taken.

Dr. McDowell

You were discussing prolactin in relationship to the corticosteroids in these fat and lean birds, and I believe you stated that prolactin was released 12 hours after the rise in corticosteroids in the fat birds versus 9 hours after the rise in corticosteroids in the lean birds. Did you measure the magnitude of the corticosteroid itself, and was there an increased level of corticosteroid in the birds where prolactin was released at 9 hours versus the 12?

Dr. Meier

Apparently not. We have measured corticosteroids by fluorescence and CBG methods. The rise of plasma corticosteroid concentration in the spring occurs near dawn and is relatively low by the time that prolactin stimulates a fattening response 12 hours later. On the other hand, prolactin can also produce a fattening response when corticosteroid levels are high. The levels of the adrenal corticoids, then, are not important. Instead, the daily rise of adrenal corticoids appears to set or entrain a series of temporal phases of responses to prolactin. I believe that the daily increase in corticosteroids sets the phases of cellular clocks and that the subsequent levels of the corticosteroids during the day are not particularly important in this respect for the regulation of fattening.

Dr. Sage

I would just like to make a comment inasmuch as I know Dr. Meier's experiments raise surprise in the eyes of people who work with mammals when they come across them for the first time. I was very dubious of these results when I first saw them and thought I would check into them perhaps a little more thoroughly. Dr. de Vlaming and I did this with two species of fish, and we got in fact much more striking results than Dr. Meier had originally reported, so we were converted. I was particularly interested in the handling effect on fat that you reported, as it seemed an obvious explanation of some of the discrepancies we were getting with different technicians doing experiments and getting different results, consistent within themselves, but differing among the individuals. Consequently, we thought there should be differences in the prolactin content of the pituitaries following release, relating to the different handling. In fact, we found that one person handling a fish will do something different with it, and subsequently the amount of prolactin that can then be assayed is different. Those who had the greatest experience in handling fish ended up with the least amount lost from the pituitary. This sort of thing adds an incredible complication to interpreting this sort of experiment on rhythms in fish.

DISCUSSION REFERENCES

Meier, A. H., Lynch, G. R., and Garcia, L. E. (1973). Daily rhythms of plasma chloride in two teleosts, *Fundulus grandis* and *Fundulus chrysotus*. Copeia 1973, 90-92.

THE ROLE OF PROLACTIN IN MAMMOGENESIS AND LACTOGENESIS

Laurence S. Jacobs

Washington University School of Medicine
Department of Medicine-Metabolism
660 S. Euclid
St. Louis, Missouri 63110

OUTLINE

I. Introduction

II. Control of Prolactin Secretion

> Hypothalamic influences
> Estrogen
> Thyroid function
> Drugs

III. Regulation of Mammary Growth and Development

> Normal hormonal requirements
> Insights gained from disease states
> Effects of pregnancy

IV. Regulation of Milk Production

> Determinants of postpartum lactation
> Relationship between serum PRL levels and lactation
> Milk PRL levels
> PRL receptor affinity
> Interactions with steroids

I. INTRODUCTION

Although a great deal of new information about the physiologic and pathologic regulation of prolactin secretion in man has become available in recent years, precise delineation of the role of prolactin in human mammogenesis and lactogenesis has been difficult. This should not be surprising in light of the fact that its role in these processes is imperfectly understood in sub-primate mammals.

Though detailed information has been accumulated on hormonal requirements for the maintenance and function of mammary explants in short-term tissue culture *in vitro*, the relevance of these observations to *in vivo* lactational physiology remains unclear. A substantial body of literature dealing with lactation and its vascular cytologic, biochemical, and physiologic aspects has been developed during the past 30 years, but many aspects of breast function remain poorly understood (Larson and Smith, 1974).

At the outset, it should be noted that many reasons for the relative paucity of our understanding of breast physiology are apparent. One of the most important of these is the large number of hormonal signals to which the breast appears to be responsive. Estrogen, progesterone, placental lactogen, and pituitary prolactin play important roles in determining breast size and in modulating breast function. Additionally, there is substantial albeit less compelling existence that lactational performance is in part dependent on normal thyroid and adrenal function; softer evidence further indicates the likelihood that the mammary gland requires insulin for normal functioning. The influence of these latter factors on normal breast development remains essentially unknown. We cannot extrapolate with very much certainty from the rodent models which have served as the basis for much of the *in vitro* information to the human lactational situation.

Because of the dominant inhibitory hypothalamic control over prolactin secretion, lesions of the stalk or hypothalamus in man which do not also totally destroy the lactotrope cell population may cause marked increases in prolactin secretion (Foley, Jacobs,

Table 1. HORMONAL FACTORS IN HUMAN MAMMARY GROWTH AND DEVELOPMENT

    I. Hormones of Established Prime Importance
        Estrogens
        Progesterone
        Prolactin
        Placental Lactogen (chorionic somatomammotropin)

   II. Hormones Probably Required in a Permissive Way
        Thyroxine/Triiodothyronine
        Insulin
        Cortisol

  III. Hormones Implicated by Animal Studies but Probably not Relevant to Human Mammogenesis
        Growth Hormone
        Aldosterone

   IV. Hormones Inhibiting Breast Development
        Androgens

Hoffman, Daughaday, and Blizzard, 1972; Snyder, Jacobs, Rabello, Sterling, Shore, Utiger, and Daughaday, 1974). One consequence of this fact is that it is hazardous to assume ablation of PRL[1] secretion following lesions of the hypothalamic-pituitary axis. Rather, empirical validation of PRL deficiency, based on radioimmunoassay measurement of circulating hormone levels, is required. Further, measurement of basal levels is insufficient. It should also be demonstrated that administration of a potent stimulus to PRL secretion such as TRH, which acts directly on the adenohypophysial lactotrope cell (Machlin, Jacobs, Cirulis, Kimes, and Miller, 1974), fails to elicit an increase in PRL secretion before one may safely conclude that hypolactotropism has been achieved. These considerations loom large when one considers the type of experimental evidence which would be required for the validation of an experimental model of PRL deficiency.

An even greater paucity of useful information exists regarding the role of prolactin in the initiation and control of mammogenesis in man. The difficulties in advancing our understanding of this problem are related primarily to the lack of a suitable experimental model. Two features contribute: first, the scarcity and expense of a suitable primate species for study; second, the technical difficulties in producing long-term isolated deficiency of prolactin without concomitantly affecting the secretion of other pituitary hormones and their target organ secretions. Nonetheless, experimental evidence supporting a major role for prolactin in animal mammogenesis is compelling (Meites and Nicoll, 1966).

In order to study the role of the hormone in mammogenesis, one should choose for study an animal in which mammary growth and development is readily identified as a normal maturational event. It would be preferable to establish a state of PRL deficiency in early postnatal life, and it would be essential of course that the PRL deficiency be an isolated one. These considerations make it difficult to draw conclusions regarding the physiologic role of prolactin in an animal, like some strains of mice, in whom growth hormone is well documented to have a potent mammotropic effect.

This brief sketch of the formidable technical barriers which have thus far impeded more rapid progress in our understanding of breast maturation and function should serve as a background for the ensuing discussion of the control of prolactin secretion. We shall return later to the question of experimental approaches to the un-

---

[1]Abbreviations used in this manuscript are: PRL: prolactin; TRH: thyrotropin releasing hormone; PIF: prolactin inhibiting factor; TSH: thyrotropin; PRH: prolactin releasing hormone; GH: growth hormone.

derstanding of human breast maturation and function.

After even the briefest consideration of some of these issues it is not hard to understand why we have yet to see a definitive experimental study of the role of prolactin in *in vivo* mammogenesis. Total ablation of adenohypophysial endocrine functions, followed by fractional replacement therapy with thyroid hormone, glucocorticoids, sex steroids, and growth hormone, might shed some light on this problem, but would be a tedious and difficult long-term experiment.

II. CONTROL OF PROLACTIN SECRETION

Unlike the remainder of the anterior pituitary hormones in man, prolactin is regulated *in vivo* by a dominant inhibitory influence of the hypothalamus. Although it is clear from a large body of experimental evidence that dopaminergic mechanisms are involved in the inhibition of PRL secretion, the major locus at which dopamine may act *in vivo* is not clear. Considerable data in animal experiments as well as in man point to an effect of dopamine to suppress PRL secretion directly from the adenohypophysis (Birge, Jacobs, Hammer, and Daughaday, 1970; Macleod and Lehmeyer, 1974; Woolf, Jacobs, Donofrio, Burday, and Schalch, 1974; Shaar and Clemens, 1974). However, the hypothalamus is very rich in dopamine (Fuxe, 1974) and this compound is found in hypophysial portal vessel blood (Ben-Jonathan, Oliver, and Mical, 1976). It is conceivable that dopaminergic mechanisms may operate *in vivo* on both the hypothalamus and the pituitary. In the clinical arena, agents which are dopamine agonists, such as the precursor L-dopa or the ergot derivative 2-α-bromoergocryptine, have been used to suppress prolactin secretion and restore menses and fertility in hyperprolactinemic-amenorrheic women (del Pozo, Varga, Wyss, Tolis, Friesen, Wenner, Vetter, and Uettwiler, 1974). At present, it is not clear whether a prolactin inhibiting factor (PIF) of peptide nature exists as a hypothalamic entity separate from dopamine or not (Shaar and Clemens, 1974).

In addition to the inhibitory effect which is readily unmasked *in vivo* by experimental transection of the pituitary stalk, evidence has accumulated that a quantitatively less important hypothalamic stimulatory effect on PRL secretion may also exist. Data in support of this concept have come from studies on avian (Nicoll, Fiorindo, McKennee, and Parsons, 1970) and porcine (Valverde and Chieffo, 1971) hypothalamus. The biochemical interpretation most appropriate to these physiologic data remain unclear, however. It has been established now for half a decade that TRH, a tripeptide of known hypothalamic residence, is a potent stimulator of PRL as well as of TSH secretion (Jacobs, Snyder, Wilbur, Utiger, and Daughaday, 1971; Bowers, Friesen, Hwang, Guyda, and Folkers, 1971). On the other hand, increasing evidence from *in vitro* pituitary incubation systems and from studies of human suckling suggests the existence of a hypothalamic factor or factors other than TRH but capable of augmenting PRL secretion. TRH can account for only a portion of the *in vitro* PRL secretion stimulable by TRH (Machlin et al., 1974), and the reflex release of PRL provoked by suckling is not accompanied by increases in serum TSH concentrations (Gautvik, Tashjian, Kourides, Weintraub, Graeber, Maloof, Suzuki, and Zuckerman, 1974). Circumstantial evidence in both rodents (Lu and Meites, 1973) and man (MacIndoe and Turkington, 1973) supports the hypothesis that neurotransmitter control of such a putative PRH might well be serotonergic rather than dopaminergic, noradrenergic, or cholinergic.

The notion that PRL may well be under dual hypothalamic control, despite the quantitative dominance of an inhibitory system, is attractive because of the lack of a known target organ signal capable of completing a closed-loop negative-feedback servo-mechanism. A similar situation may obtain as regards growth hormone, since abundant data demonstrate the dominant *in vivo* facilitatory effect of the hypothalamus on growth hormone secretion, yet this same hypothalamic tissue also contains substantial quantities of somatostatin.

A large number of hormonal and neuropharmacologic influences are capable of modifying hypothalamic control of prolactin secretion. Estrogens cause hyperplasia and probably hypertrophy of the lactotrope cells, and stimulate prolactin synthesis and secretion. This effect is dependent on both the dose and the duration of exposure of estrogens. The modest 2- to 4-fold rises in circulating estradiol-17β during pregnancy in the rhesus monkey are accompanied only by very slight increases in PRL levels (Friesen, Belanger, Guyda, and Hwang, 1972). The mammoth several hundred-fold increase in estradiol during human pregnancy is associated with a 10- to 20-fold increase in circulating prolactin (Hwang, Guyda, and Friesen, 1971; Jacobs, Mariz, and Daughaday, 1972). On the other hand, the oral administration of 5 mg of diethylstilbestrol for 1 week to normal young adult men did not raise basal serum PRL levels, but PRL responses to TRH thereafter were enhanced (Carlson, Jacobs, and Daughaday, 1973). Intermediate doses and/or durations of exposure result in intermediate results as regards PRL levels (Frantz, Kleinberg, and Noel, 1972; Yen,, Ehara, and Siler, 1974). Since only a minority of women on long-term oral contraceptives have hyperprolactinemia (Daughaday and Jacobs, 1972), however, it seems likely that considerable inter-individual variability exists in response to estrogens.

The influence of estrogens may be exerted both in the hypothalamus and directly on the pituitary as well. The precise interrelations between the effects of estrogen and of catecholamines on PRL secretion have not been delineated; nor is it certain whether the effects of estrogen are direct or mediated via neurotransmitter pathways.

Similarly, the pathways and mechanisms whereby thyroid hormone deficiency and excess affect PRL secretion are not clearly identified. Hypothyroidism is associated with augmented, and hyperthyroidism with suppressed, PRL secretion (Snyder, Jacobs, Utiger, and Daughaday, 1973). Frequently these alterations are minor in degree, so that basal levels may be normal, although significant departures of group means from those of euthyroid subjects are identified, especially in children. Stimulation with TRH reveals marked augmentation of PRL responses in hypothyroidism and suppression of responses in hyperthyroidism. Since the qualitative nature of these changes is similar to those which occur in the secretion of thyrotropin, since there is general agreement that the direct feedback effects of thyroid hormones on the pituitary are quantatively dominant in TSH feedback control, and since hyperprolactinemia unmasked by TRH occurs in both thyroidal hypothyroidism (Snyder *et al.*, 1973) and in hypothalamic hypothyroidism (Foley *et al.*, 1972), it appears that the common denominator is thyroid hormone deficiency *per se*. It further seems likely that adenohypophysial lactotrope cells have thyroid hormone receptors similar to those of the thyrotropes.

A variety of drugs have been noted to affect PRL secretion. As noted above, oral contraceptives may cause frank hyperprolactinemia in a minority of women while regular menses continue. Most often, clinically overt galactorrhea does not occur under these circumstances, probably due to the independent action of estrogens to suppress lactational responses to prolactin. The most common drug-related abnormality of PRL secretion is that which occurs after cessation of oral contraceptive therapy. The relatively common post-pill amenorrhea, in which continued gonadotropin suppression continues inappropriately after cessation of therapy, is on occasion accompanied by hyperprolactinemia, with or without galactorrhea. These clinical manifestations may represent a functional hypothalamic disturbance, or they may herald the presence of a prolactin-secreting pituitary adenoma brought to the threshold of clinical detection by the challenge of oral contraceptive therapy.

Other drugs which may cause hyperprolactinemia or galactorrhea do so either by depleting the hypothalamus of catecholamines or by interfering with aminergic transmission in the hypothalamus. Reserpine is the prototype of the former action, and alphamethyldopa, phenothiazines, and butyrophenones interfere with receptor recognition of dopamine. As with oral contraceptives, the overt clinical manifestations--oligomenorrhea or amenorrhea coupled with galactorrhea--probably represent only those individuals with the most marked chemical abnormalities, the tip of the clinical iceberg. With phenothiazines, for example, the overwhelming majority of people taking significantly more than 50 mg/day equivalent of chlorpromazine will be found to be hyperprolactinemic, yet only a minority will have irregular or absent menses, or galactorrhea. These drugs probably act by limiting the secretion of PIF or by suppressing its action.

III. REGULATION OF MAMMARY GROWTH AND DEVELOPMENT

Our current understanding of the normal sequence of maturational and gestational growth and development of the mammary gland of necessity derives primarily from studies carried out in small laboratory rodents and in dairy animals. Not all the conclusions suggested by these data have been validated in primates.

There is general agreement that maturational growth of the mammary gland is probably directly related to prevailing secretory rates of estrogen *in vivo*. *In vitro*, the two hormones required for growth and cell division in preparation for prolactin induced milk secretion are insulin and hydrocortisone. In some strains of mice, growth hormone is potently mammotropic (Nandi and Bern, 1961), but human and monkey GH appear to be unique among growth hormones in having lactogenic and mammotropic properties not accountable on the basis of contamination by prolactin. Bovine and ovine GH's are not lactogenic.

In organ culture of mouse mammary gland, aldosterone appears to be capable of stimulating ductal differentiation and branching in glands pretreated with insulin and prolactin (Ceriani, 1970), although critical *in vivo* testing of the need for aldosterone in normal mammogenesis has not been done. No detailed studies of hormonal changes during puberty in experimental animals appear to have been carried out at present.

In humans, though *in vitro* organ culture data are lacking, there is a good deal of information on levels of prolactin and of other potentially relevant hormones at various ages and stages of pubertal and gestational breast development. In addition, a number of hormonally defined disease processes may shed light on the questions at hand.

Estrogens stimulate mammary gland hyperplasia in man. Like other estrogen effects, this response is dependent on both the estrogen effects; this response is dependent on both the estrogen level and the duration of tissue exposure to it. Alveolar proliferation, which occurs post-pubertally and is intensified during pregnancy, is highly dependent upon the adequacy of progesterone secretion. It seems reasonable to infer from the organ culture data that normality of cortisol and insulin secretion may be prerequisites for normal mammary growth and development. No systematic clinical data collection on breast development in pubertal girls with Addison's disease has been done, to my knowledge, and juvenile diabetics are treated of course with insulin. Hence, we may have to be satisfied with guesses and inferences in this matter. It further seems quite likely that euthyroidism may be yet another prerequisite for fully normal breast development.

The role played by prolactin in mammogenesis in humans remains unclear. Circulating levels of prolactin are only slightly higher in adult women of reproductive age than in men, and measurements in prepubertal children have generally given results comparable to those in men (Foley et al., 1972; Guyda and Friesen, 1973). In cross-sectional studies of puberty, the observed rise in PRL levels seemed to be gradual (Guyda and Friesen, 1973). Similarly, the rise in estradiol levels appears to be gradual during puberty, with achievement of adult female levels only late in the pubertal process (Ehara, Yen, and Siler, 1975), whereas breast budding and major breast growth in girls are relatively early pubertal events.

These data do not support the concept that major changes in estrogen or prolactin levels are responsible for human mammogenesis. Rather, it seems likely that subtle changes in hormonal secretion, coupled with alterations in mammary responsiveness to the hormonal milieu, may be responsible for human pubertal breast growth. It seems reasonable to assume that certain minimal levels of prolactin may be required, in a permissive way, for breast development to occur under the influence of sex steroids.

The occurrence of hypopituitarism or hypogonadism prepubertally is associated with deficient mammary development in the absence of replacement therapy. In hypopituitary girls, treatment with glucocorticoids, thyroid hormone, and growth hormone does not result in notable mammary development. This requires treatment with estrogen, estrogen plus progesterone, or gonadotropins. Prolactin secretion is frequently normal in hypopituitary subjects. In girls with Turner's syndrome, breast development requires sex steroid therapy. Women with isolated growth hormone deficiency develop normal breasts and are fully capable of normal postpartum lactational performance (Tyson, Hwang, Guyda, and Friesen, 1972; Rimoin, Holzman, Merimee, Rabinowitz, Barnes, Tyson, and McKusick, 1968).

These considerations strongly suggest that in humans, although eucorticism and euthyroidism may be required for the full expression of mammary growth, maturation, and lactational function, they exert a permissive role only. Growth hormone appears not to play an important role. Since most early breast growth is accounted for by ductal proliferation without much alveolar budding in normal girls whose aldosterone secretion is adequate, one may also question the relevance of the mouse mammary organ culture data cited above to the normal human situation.

Although systematic observations in man on the role of androgens in mammary development have not been made, it is clear from clinical observations in women with virilizing syndromes and in men with alcoholism and gynecomastia that androgens act in opposition to estrogens as regards breast development. No comparison of PRL levels or estradiol levels between buxom and flat-chested women have been made. Table 1 lists the hormones which may be involved in mammary growth and development.

The growth and development of the breast during pregnancy is accounted for by the combined effects of hypersecretion of estrogens, progesterone, prolactin, and chorionic somatomammotropin. Considerable alveolar hypertrophy occurs during pregnancy, and if it were not for the inhibitory effect of very high circulating estrogens on the breast response to mammotropic hormones, undoubtedly copious lactation would be a regular feature of the third trimester of pregnancy. As it is, the hormonal bombardment of the breast in late pregnancy is quite remarkable; estradiol and progesterone levels are several hundred-fold higher in late pregnancy than in the follicular phase of the menstrual cycle. Chorionic somatomammotropin levels may rise as high as 10-12 µg/ml, several orders of magnitude higher than the usual circulating levels of other peptide hormones of comparable molecular weight. Pituitary prolactin levels, under the influence of estrogens, average about 200 ng/ml at term, or roughly twenty times higher than nonpregnant levels.

IV. REGULATION OF MILK PRODUCTION

I will not review here the extensive literature on regulation of lactation in dairy animals, but will rather focus on what is known regarding this subject in women. Many of the same hormonal influences important in the regulation of mammary growth and development play prominent roles in the control of lactation. Failure of lactation in otherwise endocrinologically normal women has been described in association with isolated deficiency of prolactin (Turkington, 1972); these data were obtained by PRL bioassay measurement following administration of phenothiazines, and have yet to be confirmed. From the *in vitro* organ culture experience, one may suspect that normal insulin secretion, eucorticism, and euthyroidism are important permissive prerequisites for normal lactation. The secretory apparatus must have reached some minimal threshold stage of development under the influence of estrogen and progesterone. Induction of milk protein synthesis is dependent on the mammotropic hormones prolactin or chorionic somatomammotropin. The secretion of milk following all this hormonal preparation further depends on withdrawal of estrogen and progesterone, as well as on intact mechanisms for oxytocin release and myoepithelial basket cell contraction. Tactile stimulation of the breast and nipple results in reflex release of PRL (Kolodny, Jacobs, and Daughaday, 1972; Noel, Suh, and Frantz, 1974) and of oxytocin as well. In endocrinologically normal but nonpregnant women, lactogenesis can be induced by administration of estrogen and a regular program of tactile manipulation of the breast and nipple, followed by abrupt cessation of the estrogen treatment and a waiting period of a few days (Tyson, Khojandi, Huth, and Andreasson, 1975). Similarly, there is a normal delay of several days following delivery before milk secretion becomes well established postpartum. The important factors responsible for this delay include time required to escape from the inhibition previously exercised by high levels of estrogen and progesterone.

With delivery of the placenta, the source of all the placental lactogen (chorionic somatomammotropin) and the great bulk of the progesterone and estrogen produced during late pregnancy is removed. Circulating levels of these hormones fall in accord with their respective half-lives in the serum, but the secretion of prolactin does not change nearly as rapidly. Even in nonbreast-feeding mothers experiencing no suckling stimulus, it may take 2 to 3 weeks for basal prolactin levels to return to nonpregnant levels. This indicates substantial temporal persistence of the estrogen stimulation after its removal, and is consistent with the duration of other biological actions of estrogens. In breast-feeding mothers, the decline of PRL levels is substantially slowed, and nonpregnant fasting levels may not be reached for several weeks. Table 2 summarizes the factors involved in the initiation of postpartum lactation.

As has been shown, suckling episodes result in dramatic rises in serum PRL levels during the early puerperium (Tyson *et al.*, 1972). Later during lactation, the serum PRL either increases much less sharply with suckling, or in some cases may not rise measurably at all; basal PRL levels are normal. Although there is some variation in serum PRL from moment to moment, especially in hyperprolactinemic states (Jacobs and Daughaday, 1973), there is reason to believe that randomly obtained levels may nonetheless reflect integrated 24-hour levels reasonably well (Malarkey, 1975). Thus normal lactation seems to proceed quite well in the absence of accelerated PRL secretion. At the same time, most breast-feeding women remain amenorrheic or oligomenorrheic and rather severely estrogen-deficient. Nonpuerperal galactorrhea is also frequently associated with hypoestrogenism and menstrual irregularities or amenorrhea. Thus, in contrast to breast development, which requires estrogen, lactation seems to require suppression or removal of estrogen. Further, it would appear that

Table 2. FACTORS INVOLVED IN THE INITIATION OF POSTPARTUM LACTATION

    Postpartum Time Lag
    Rapidly Falling Estrogens
    Rapidly Falling Progesterone
    Tactile Stimulation of the
     Breast and Nipple

Table 3. ASSESSMENT OF PROLACTIN EFFECTS ON THE BREAST

Single Determinations *vs*. Secretory Rates
Subtle alterations Maintained over Months or Years
Synergistic Effects of Multiple Hormones
Variations in Mammary Response to the Hormonal Milieu
Systemic *vs*. Mammary Hormone Concentrations

more PRL is required for the initiation of lactation than for its maintenance. Table 3 indicates some of the considerations which need to be kept in mind as one tries to relate measured PRL levels to breast function.

The possibility does of course exist that the measured serum PRL level is not an accurate reflection of the hormonal milieu to which the breast is exposed. In order to assess this possibility, and because the presence of immunoreactive PRL in milk had been reported in experimental animals (McMurtry and Malvern, 1974a, 1974b), we have measured the PRL in simultaneously obtained milk and serum specimens in a series of women with nonpuerperal galactorrhea. Figure 1 shows the systematic gradient which exists between these two fluids, the prolactin concentration in milk being significantly higher than that found in serum. Thus the breast does to a certain extent act as a concentrating mechanism. Whether the PRL in milk which is immunologically intact is a more valid index of the hormonal exposure of milk-secreting cells than that in serum remains to be shown, however. Although the mechanism by which apparently intact prolactin finds its say into milk is not known, it seems clear that the hormone must traverse the capillary side of the alveolar cell plasma membrane, the cell interior, and the luminal or ductular surface plasma membrane as well. Cell penetrance by polypeptide hormones such as prolactin has in the past been thought not to occur in relation to hormone action; however, recently intracellular polypeptide hormone receptors have been tentatively identified (Posner and Bergeron, 1976) and such a mechanism may be involved in the transfer of prolactin from serum to milk. A similar gradient in PRL seems to exist in postpartum lactating women, so this mechanism is not restricted to situations of abnormal pathophysiology.

It is a reasonably frequent occurrence ot find normal PRL levels in the serum of women with nonpuerperal galactorrhea of diverse etiologies. This is especially common in women in whom regular menses persist despite galactorrhea, and no apparent cause for the lactation can be found. Several possible explanations exist for continued galactorrhea despite normal PRL levels. One may postulate that during the early phases of the disorder, higher levels of PRL may have prevailed while lactation was being established.

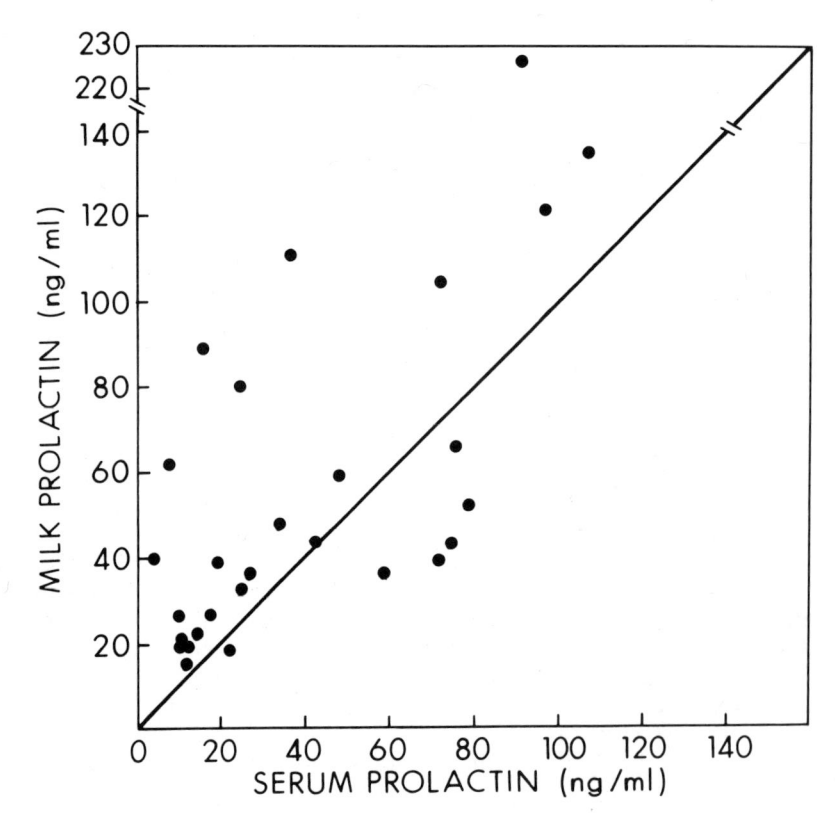

Figure 1. Correlation between serum PRL levels and simultaneously obtained milk PRL levels in women with nonpuerperal galactorrhea. The bulk of the data points fall above the diagonal line of identity, indicating a systematic gradient from milk to serum. Whether enhanced entry into, or diminished clearance from milk is the prime factor responsible for the higher milk PRL levels is not known.

Table 4. FACTORS CAPABLE OF INFLUENCING MAMMARY RESPONSIVITY TO PROLACTIN

    I. PRE-RECEPTOR EVENTS
        Prior Hormonal Milieu

   II. THE PROLACTIN RECEPTOR
        Affinity
        Capability

  III. POST-RECEPTOR EVENTS
        Coupling of Hormone Binding to Adenylate Cyclase
        Protein Kinase
        Phosphorylation of Intracellular Proteins
        K_m, V_{max}, of Enzymes Involved in Milk Fat and/or Carbohydrate Synthesis

Alternatively, one may explain such a situation by the suggestion that milk PRL levels may be higher than those in serum, as shown in Figure 1. Finally, an altered, heightened tissue responsivity to PRL could account for such findings. One way in which heightened tissue sensitivity may be explained is by an increase in either the number or the affinity of hormone receptors. Figure 2 demonstrates that just such an increase in PRL affinity does in fact occur in rabbit mammary glands during postpartum lactation. Individual Scatchard plots of PRL to representative early (first postpartum week) and last (just prior to weaning) mammary gland membrane preparations are shown. Although the mechanism responsible for this 2.5-fold increase in PRL receptor affinity is not known, such as increase could help account for continued lactation in the face of falling serum PRL levels. Table 4 indicates that changes in hormone receptor affinity represent only one of several possible mechanisms which might underlie enhanced tissue responsivity.

On occasion, despite very high serum PRL levels, sometimes in the thousands of nanograms per ml, no mammary manifestations attributable to hyperprolactinemia may occur. This type of dissociation between clinical manifestations and hormone overproduction is most often seen in patients harboring pituitary adenomas. The absence of gynecomastia in such men, and of galactorrhea in such women, is

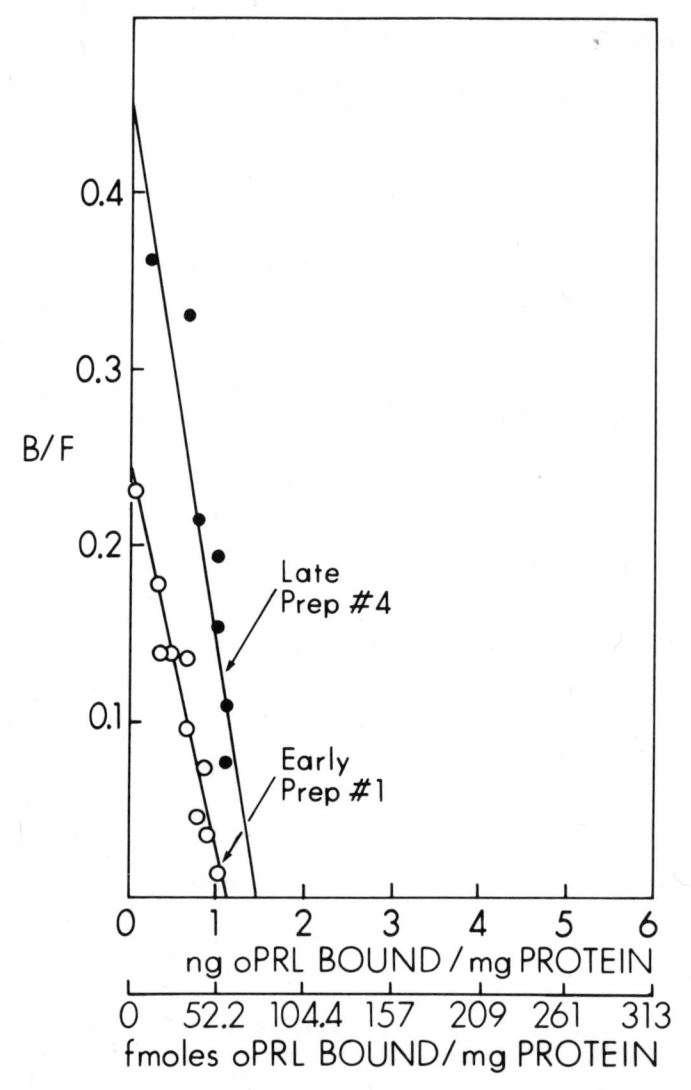

Figure 2. Scatchard plots of the interaction of single representative early (first postpartum week) and late (immediately prior to weaning) mammary receptor preps with iodinated ovine prolactin. The binding capacity of the two preparations is similar (60 and 76 fmoles/mg protein) but the affinity of the late prep is 3.8-fold greater than that of the early prep (K_a, 1 x $10^{10} M^{-1}$ *vs.* 2.6 x $10^9 M^{-1}$).

most satisfactorily explained by postulating that the frequently present hypogonadism results in hypoestrogenism and breasts which are less sensitive to the actions of PRL. Most men with PRL-secreting pituitary adenomas who do have galactorrhea exhibit serum PRL levels which are very markedly elevated, often in excess of 1000 ng/ml. Although many women with such tumors and galactorrhea have PRL levels which are only modestly elevated, suggesting that the clinical expression of hyperprolactinemia at the breast is facilitated by estrogens, nonetheless men with such tumors occasionally have galactorrhea with PRL levels less than 100 ng/ml. Uniformly these men are found to be hypogonadal. Thus it would seem, as in cirrhotics with gynecomastia, that breast responses to sex steroids and to PRL appear to depend on the estrogen/androgen ratio more than the absolute level of either.

REFERENCES

Ben-Jonathan, N., Oliver, C, and Mical, R.S. (1976). Dopamine secretion into hypophysial portal blood during the estrus cycle and pregnancy in the rat. Program, 58th Meeting, Endocrine Society, Abstract 269, Endocrinology 98, Supplement, p. 191.

Birge, C.A., Jacobs, L.S., Hammer, C.T., and Daughaday, W.H. (1970). Catecholamine inhibition of prolactin secretion by isolated rat adenohypophyses. Endocrinology 86, 120-130.

Bowers, C.Y., Friesen, H.G., Hwang, P., Guyda, H.J., and Folkers, K. (1971). Prolactin and thyrotropin release in man by synthetic pyroglutamyl-histidyl-prolinamide. Biochem. Biophys. Res. Commun. 45, 1033-1041.

Carlson, H.E., Jacobs, L.S., and Daughaday, W.H. (1973). Growth hormone, thyrotropin and prolactin responses to thyrotropin-releasing hormone following diethylstilbestrol pretreatment. J. Clin. Endocrinol. Metab. 37, 488-490.

Ceriani, R.L. (1970) Fetal mammary gland differentiation *in vitro* in response to hormones. I. Morphological findings. Developm. Biol. 21, 506-529.

Daughaday, W.H. and Jacobs, L.S. (1972). Normal and pathologic secretion of prolactin in man. In: *Endocrinology*, Proceedings IV International Congress of Endocrinology (Scow, R.O., ed.), pp. 622-628, Excerpta Medica International Congress Series No. 273.

del Pozo, E., Varga, L., Wyss, H., Tolis, G., Friesen, H., Wenner, R., Vetter, L., and Uettwiler, A. (1974). Clinical and hormonal response to bromocriptin (CB-154) in the galactorrhea syndromes. J. Clin. Endocrinol. Metab. 39, 18-36.

Ehara, Y., Yen, S.S.C., and Siler, T.M. (1975). Serum prolactin levels during puberty. Amer. J. Obstet. Gynec. 121, 995-997.

Foley, T.P. Jr., Jacobs, L.S., Hoffman, W., Daughaday, W.H., and Blizzard, R.M. (1972). Human prolactin and thyrotropin concentrations in the serums of normal and hypopituitary children before and after the administration of synthetic thyrotropin-releasing hormone. J. Clin. Invest. 51, 2143-2150.

Frantz, A.G., Kleinberg, D.L., and Noel, G.L. (1972). Studies on prolactin in man. Rec. Prog. Horm. Res. 28, 527-590.

Friesen, H.G., Belanger, C., Guyda, H.J., and Hwang, P. (1972). The synthesis and secretion of placental lactogen and pituitary prolactin. In: *Lactogenic Hormones* (Wolstenholme, G.F.W. and Knight, J., eds.), pp. 83-103, Churchill-Livingstone, London.

Fuxe, K. (1964). Cellular localization of monoamines in the median eminence and the infundibular stem of some mammals. Z. Zellforsch Mikrosk. Anat. 61, 710-724.

Gautvik, K.M., Tashjian, A.H. Jr., Kourides, I.A., Weintraub, B.D., Graeber, C.T., Maloof, F., Suzuki, K., and Zuckerman, J.E. (1974). Thyrotropin-releasing hormone is not the sole physiologic mediator of prolactin release during suckling. New Engl. J. Med. 290, 1162-1165.

Hwang, P., Guyda, H., and Friesen, H. (1971). A radioimmunossay for human prolactin. Proc. Natl. Acad. Sci. 68, 1902-1906.

Jacobs, L.S. and Daughaday, W.H. (1973). Pathophysiology and control of prolactin secretion in patients with pituitary and hypothalamic disease. In: *Human Prolactin* (Pasteels, J.L. and Robyn, C., eds.), pp. 189, International Congress Series No. 308, Excerpta Medica, Amsterdam.

Jacobs, L.S., Mariz, I.K., and Daughaday, W.H. (1972). A mixed heterologous radioimmunoassay for human prolactin. J. Clin. Endocrinol. Metab. 34, 484-490.

Jacobs, L.S., Snyder, P.J., Wilber, J.F., Utiger, R.D., and Daughaday, W.H. (1971). Increased serum prolactin after administration of synthetic thyrotropin releasing hormone (TRH) in man. J. Clin. Endocrinol. Metab. 33, 996-999.

Kolodny, R.C., Jacobs, L.S., and Daughaday, W.A. (1972). Mammary stimulation causes prolactin secretion in non-lactating women. Nature 238, 284-286.

Larson, B.L. and Smith, V.R., eds. (1974). *Lactation/A Comprehensive Treatise*, 3 volumes, Academic Press. Volume 1: *The Mammary Gland/Development and Maintenance*, Volume 2: *Biosynthesis and Secretion of Milk/Diseases*, and Volume 3: *Nutrition and Biochemistry of Milk/Maintenance of Lactation*.

Lu, K.H. and Meites, J. (1973). Effects of serotonin precursors and melatonin on serum prolactin release in rats. Endocrinology 93, 152-155.

Machlin, L.J., Jacobs, L.S., Cirulis, N., Kimes, R., and Miller, R. (1974). An assay for growth hormone and prolactin-releasing activities using a bovine pituitary cell culture system. Endocrinology 95, 1350-1358.

MacIndoe, J.H. and Turkington, R.W. (1973). Stimulation of human prolactin secretion by intravenous infusion of L-tryptophan. J. Clin. Invest. 52, 1972-1978.

Macleod, R.M. and Lehmeyer, J.E. (1974). Studies on the mechanisms of the dopamine-mediated inhibition of prolactin secretion. Endocrinology 94, 1077-1085.

Malarkey, W.B. (1975). Nonpuerperal lactation and normal prolactin regulation. J. Clin. Endocrinol. Metab. 40, 198-204.

McMurtry, J.P. and Malven, P.V. (1974a). Radioimmunoassay of endogenous and exogenous prolactin in milk of rats. J. Endocrinol. 61, 211-217.

McMurtry, J.P. and Malven, P.V. (1974b). Experimental alterations of prolactin levels in goat milk and blood plasma. Endocrinology 95, 559-564.

Meites, J. and Nicoll, C.S. (1966). Adenohypophysis: Prolactin. Ann. Rev. Physiol. 28, 57-88.

Nandi, S. and Bern, H.A. (1961). The hormone responsible for lactogenesis in BALB-cCrgl mice. Gen. Comp. Endocrinol. 1, 195-210.

Nicoll, C.S., Fiorindo, R.P., McKennee, C.R., and Parsons, J.A. (1970). Assay of hypothalamic factors which regulate prolactin secretion. In: *Hypophysiotropic Hormones of the Hypothalamus: Assay and Chemistry* (Meites, J., ed.), pp. 115-144, Williams and Wilkins, Baltimore.

Noel, G.L., Suh, H.K., and Frantz, A.G. (1974). Prolactin release during nursing and breast stimulation in postpartum and non-postpartum subjects. J. Clin. Endocrinol. Metab. 38, 413-423.

Posner, B.I. and Bergeron, J.J.M. (1976). Intracellular polypeptide hormone receptors. Program, 58th Meeting, Endocrine Society, Abstract 218, Endocrinology 98, Supplement, pp. 165.

Rimoin, D.L., Holzman, G.B., Merimee, T.J., Rabinowitz, D., Barnes, A.C., Tyson, J.E., and McKusick, V.A. (1968). Lactation in the absence of human growth hormone. J. Clin. Endocrinol. Metab. 28, 1183-1188.

Shaar, C.J. and Clemens, J.A. (1974). The role of catecholamines in the release of anterior pituitary prolactin *in vitro*. Endocrinology 95, 1201-1212.

Snyder, P.J., Jacobs, L.S., Utiger, R.D., and Daughaday, W.H. (1973). Thyroid hormone inhibition of the prolactin response to thyrotropin-releasing hormone. J. Clin. Invest. 52, 2324-2329.

Snyder, P.J., Jacobs, L.S., Rabello, M.M., Sterling, F.H., Shore, R.N., Utiger, R.D., and Daughaday, W.H. (1974). Diagnostic value of thyrotropin-releasing hormone in pituitary and hypothalamic diseases: Assessment of thyrotropin and prolactin secretion in 100 patients. Annals Int. Med. 81, 751-757.

Turkington, R.W. (1972). Phenothiazine stimulation test for prolactin reserve: The syndrome of isolated prolactin deficiency. J. Clin. Endocrinol. Metab. 34, 247-250.

Tyson, J.E., Hwang, P., Guyda, H., and Friesen, H.G. (1972). Studies of prolactin secretion in human pregnancy. Amer. J. Obstet. Gynecol. 113, 14-20.

Tyson, J.E., Khojandi, M., Huth, J., and Andreasson, B. (1975). The influence of prolactin secretion on human lactation. J. Clin. Endocrinol. Metab. 40, 764-773.

Valverde, C., and Chieffo, V. (1971). Prolactin releasing factors in porcine hypothalamic extracts. Program, 53rd Meeting, Endocrine Society, Abstract 83, Endocrinology 88, Supplement, p. A84.

Woolf, P.D., Jacobs, L.S., Donofrio, R., Burday, S.Z., and Schalch, D.S. (1974). Secondary hypopituitarism: Evidence for continuing regulation of hormone release. J. Clin. Endocrinol. Metab. 38, 71-76.

Yen, S.S.C., Ehara, Y., and Siler, T.M. (1974). Augmentation of prolactin secretion by estrogen in hypogonadal women. J. Clin. Invest. 53, 652-655.

DISCUSSION AFTER DR. JACOBS' PAPER

Dr. Barnawell

I wonder if you know of any measurements of prolactin levels during the menstrual cycle.

Dr. Jacobs

Yes, several groups of investigators have measured prolactin levels in a very large number of normally cycling women. Although one group of European investigators claim that there is a significant increase in prolactin during the luteal phase, I think by and large most investigators have found no significant differences, so I would say that there is no significant variation in prolactin during the menstrual cycle.

Dr. Barnawell

Except for the possibility that nocturnal levels might be higher.

Dr. Jacobs

Yes, that remains a possibility.

Dr. Klein

Dr. Yen published data which showed that the nocturnal rise in prolactin at approximately mid-cycle is about twice as high as during either the follicular or luteal phase, but that's on only one patient (Ehara, Siler, Vandenberg, Sinha, and Yen, 1973). Has anyone investigated the biological activity of the prolactin found in some of the patients with tumors who don't lactate? Could this be immunoassayable prolactin that is not biologically active?

Dr. Jacobs

Some of the best data on this question were shown by Dr. Frantz in terms of the good general correlation between bioassay and radioimmunoassay results. In addition, Dr. Friesen has shown excellent correlation between radioimmunoassay and radioreceptor assay results in a large number of specimens spanning both the physiologic and pharmacologic ranges (Friesen, 1973). These data suggest strongly that the failure to observe lactation in many women with prolactin-producing pituitary adenomas is the result of variable breast responses rather than biologically inactive hormone.

Dr. Sage

I'm not familiar with the clinical literature, but the La Leche league reports on a number of cases of women who have never had children, but who adopt children and are capable of producing milk. Have any of these been followed clinically and the prolactin levels assayed?

Dr. Jacobs

Not to my knowledge. It is well documented, however, that postmenopausal grandmothers have successfully suckled their grandchildren. This used to be common in certain African tribal communities in which the men hunted and the reproductive age women did all the agricultural field work. The critical factor here, and in the La Leche reports to which you refer, is probably tactile stimulation of the breast and especially the nipple. Such tactile stimulation can, reflexly, cause release of prolactin. The reflex appears to be estrogen-sensitive.

I might add a fascinating bit of what one might call "mammaryology" in the marsupial. Kangaroos not infrequently give birth while still breastfeeding, and it is not unusual, I understand, for the rather advanced joey at age one or more to be breastfeeding at the same time that there is a newborn in the pouch breastfeeding. It has been shown that the composition of the milk produced by the two teats is markedly different. There are differences in protein electrophoretic patterns and differences in fat composition. Since they come from the same mother, one would presume that the hormonal milieu is the same. Hence, the observed differences in composition may relate to differences in quantity, quality, or frequency of the tactile stimulation produced by the neonate and that of the joey.

DISCUSSION REFERENCES

Ehara, Y., Siler, T., Vandenberg, G., Sinha, Y.M., and Yen, S.S.C. (1973). Circulating prolactin levels during the menstrual cycle: Episodic release and diurnal variation. Amer. J. Obstet. Gynec. 117, 962-970.

Friesen, H.G. (1973). In *Human Prolactin* (Pasteels, J.L. and Robyn, C., eds.), ICS #308, Excerpta Medica, Amsterdam.

INHIBITION OF THE RENAL RESPONSE TO INTRAVENOUS PROLACTIN BY ADH

G.C. Bond, J.N. Pasley, T.I. Koike, and L. Llerena

Department of Physiology and Biophysics
University of Arkansas Medical Center
Little Rock, AR   72201

The injection of ovine prolactin intramuscularly in conscious human subjects (Horrobin, Lloyd, Lipton, Burstyn, Durkin, and Muiruri, 1971) or intraperitoneally in conscious rats (Lockett and Nail, 1965) has been shown to produce an antidiuresis and antinatriuresis which persists for several hours. The duration of the renal response both in the human subjects and in the rats was due partially to the route of prolactin administration. Thus, to define more clearly the time course of the renal response to prolactin we have monitored renal function in rats before and after the intravenous injection of prolactin.

Male Sprague-Dawley rats were anesthetized with pentobarbital (50 mg/kg). A cannula was inserted in the trachea and a jugular vein catheterized. A polyvinyl catheter (2 cm in length) was inserted into the fundus of the bladder and tied securely in place. The animals were placed in the ventral position on a table inside an infant incubator which was maintained at 33°C and 75% relative humidity. A solution of 0.45% sodium chloride and 2.5% dextrose was infused through the jugular catheter at a rate of 0.15 ml/min. Urine was allowed to drop through an electronic drop counter into tared tubes. A relatively stable urine flow was established and after two 15-minute control collection periods an injection of 20 µg of ovine prolactin (NIH SP10) dissolved in 0.2 ml of saline was injected through the jugular catheter. A group of control rats received an intravenous injection of 0.2 ml of saline without the prolactin. Sodium and potassium concentrations in urine were determined by flame photometry and urinary osmolality by freezing point depression. The Mann-Whitney U test (two-tailed) was used to compare statistically the renal responses produced by the intravenous injections of prolactin and saline.

Table 1 shows a comparison of the effects of prolactin and saline on urine flow and urinary osmolality. Injections were made immediately after the urine collection at time 0. During the first 15-minute post-injection collection period urine flow decreased and urine osmolality increased in the prolactin-injected rats. These changes were statistically significant. The three remaining collection periods showed no significant differences in either flow or osmolality. The records obtained from the drop counter indicated that urine flow began to decrease approximately one minute after injection of prolactin and then returned to control levels within 15 minutes. Table 2 indicates that the intravenous injection of prolactin produced no statistically significant changes in either the excretion of sodium or the excretion of potassium.

Table 1. THE EFFECT OF PROLACTIN ON URINE FLOW AND URINARY OSMOLALITY IN NORMAL RATS

	n	Urine Flow (% of control) time in minutes -15, 0, 15, 30, 45, 60	Osmolality (% of control) time in minutes -15, 0, 15, 30, 45, 60
Saline	6	101 99 117 108 87 95 ±1 ±1 ±10 ±12 ±6 ±11	101 99 103 100 128 138 ±1 ±1 ±10 ±23 ±15 ±20
Prolactin	8	100 100 74 88 90 97 ±1 ±1 ±4 ±5 ±4 ±9	102 98 137 117 117 121 ±2 ±2 ±8 ±11 ±11 ±8
p		.001	.001

Values as means and their standard errors

Table 2. THE EFFECT OF PROLACTIN ON SODIUM EXCRETION AND POTASSIUM EXCRETION IN NORMAL RATS

	n	Urine Flow (% of control) time in minutes -15, 0, 15, 30, 45, 60	Osmolality (% of control) time in minutes -15, 0, 15, 30, 45, 60
Saline	6	102 99 149 142 164 188 ±3 ±3 ±20 ±23 ±78 ±27	103 98 125 126 137 150 ±3 ±3 ±8 ±10 ±12 ±25
Prolactin	8	100 100 132 142 156 197 ±3 ±3 ±15 ±21 ±22 ±35	98 102 126 133 148 224 ±3 ±3 ±9 ±19 ±22 ±45
p			

Values as means and their standard errors

The decrease in urine flow and increase in urine osmolality which occurred during the 15-minute collection period after injection of prolactin suggests that the clearance of free water by the kidney had been diminished. This effect of prolactin on renal function, therefore, is similar to the effect which is observed following the intravenous injection of antidiuretic hormone (ADH). Consequently, we performed an additional series of experiments to examine the possibility that maximum antidiuretic doses of circulating ADH could prevent the renal response to prolactin. Rats were treated as described above with the exception that pitressin was added to the infusion solution so that each rat received 60 µU of ADH per minute per 100 grams of body weight throughout the experiment (Atherton, Evans, Green, and Thomas, 1971). After stabilization of urine flow 20 µg of prolactin were given intravenously. A control group of rats which was infused with the same dose of pitressin was injected intravenously with 0.2 ml of saline without prolactin.

Table 3 compares the effects of an intravenous injection of prolactin to the effects of saline on urine flow and urinary osmolality in ADH-loaded rats. Note that in the prolactin-injected rats high circulating levels of ADH blocked the decrease in urine flow and increase in osmolality observed previously in the normal rats during the first 15-minute post-injected collection period. There was, however, an increase in urine flow at 45 minutes. As shown in Table 4 there also was a statistically significant increase in sodium excretion 45 minutes after injection of prolactin. It is likely, therefore, that the increase in urine flow was secondary to the increase in sodium excretion. No statistically significant changes occurred in the excretion of potassium.

Table 3. THE EFFECT OF PROLACTIN ON URINE FLOW AND URINARY OSMOLALITY IN ADH-LOADED RATS

	n	Urine Flow (% of control) time in minutes -15 0 15 30 45 60	Osmolality (% of control) time in minutes -15 0 15 30 45 60
Saline	8	99 102 117 123 110 115 ±1 ±1 ±6 ±10 ±6 ±9	102 98 92 91 90 88 ±1 ±1 ±1 ±3 ±2 ±3
Prolactin	7	100 100 110 128 132 131 ±1 ±1 ±6 ±8 ±6 ±9	101 99 94 88 85 81 ±1 ±1 ±3 ±3 ±2 ±4
p		.02	

Values represent means and their standard error

Table 4. THE EFFECT OF PROLACTIN ON SODIUM EXCRETION AND POTASSIUM EXCRETION IN ADH-LOADED RATS

	n	\multicolumn{6}{c}{Sodium Excretion (% of control) time in minutes}	\multicolumn{6}{c}{Potassium Excretion (% of control) time in minutes}
		-15	0	15	30	45	60	-15	0	15	30	45	60
Saline	8	100 ±1	100 ±1	110 ±4	114 ±7	103 ±4	104 ±7	100 ±1	100 ±1	92 ±6	92 ±6	102 ±5	103 ±11
Prolactin	7	100 ±1	100 ±1	108 ±6	123 ±6	124 ±5	128 ±10	103 ±1	97 ±1	88 ±5	96 ±6	91 ±5	88 ±7
p					.01								

Values represent means and their standard errors

In summary, the intravenous injection of 20 µg of ovine prolactin in normal rats produces a decrease in urine flow and an increase in urinary osmolality without affecting the renal excretion of sodium and potassium. The response lasted for approximately 15 minutes and could be blocked by the presence of high circulating levels of ADH. These results suggest that prolactin may produce an effect of renal function by causing an increase in the release of ADH from the posterior pituitary or by acting at the same site in the renal tubule as ADH.

REFERENCES

Horrobin, D.F., Lloyd, I.J., Lipton, A., Burstyn, P.G., Durkin, N., and Muiruri, K.L. (1971). Actions of prolactin on human renal function. Lancet ii, 352-354.

Lockett, M.F. and Nail, B. (1965). A comparative study of the renal actions of growth and lactogenic hormones in rats. J. Physiol. 180, 147-156.

Atherton, J.C., Evans, J.A., Green, R., and Thomas, S. (1971). Influence of variations in hydration and in solute excretion on the effects of lysine-vasopressin infusion on urinary and renal composition in the conscious rat. J. Physiol. 213, 311-327.

The prolactin used in this experiment was kindly supplied by the National Institute of Arthritis and Metabolic Disease.

This study was supported in part by Grant HL 16303 from the National Institutes of Health.

THE EFFECT OF ADRENALECTOMY ON THE RENAL RESPONSE TO INTRAVENOUS PROLACTIN

J.N. Pasley, G.C. Bond, T.I. Koike, and L. Llerena

Department of Physiology and Biophysics
University of Arkansas Medical Center
Little Rock, AR 72201

The possibility has been suggested that prolactin may interact with adrenal hormones to affect renal function in addition to the evidence indicating a direct effect on the kidney. Burstyn, Horrobin, and Manku (1972) and Horrobin, Manku, and Burstyn (1973) have shown that aldosterone can induce a natriuresis in the presence of excess salt intake or excess cortisol and that this natriuresis can be reversed by prolactin injection. Moreover, Relkin and Adachi (1973) have suggested that prolactin is necessary for the enhanced aldosterone secretion rates observed in sodium-deprived rats. These studies indicated that prolactin must be present, at least under certain conditions, in order for aldosterone to induce an antinatriuretic effect. Whether aldosterone is necessary for prolactin to affect kidney function is not known. An experiment was designed, therefore, to determine if the adrenals, i.e. aldosterone, must be present for the renal effects of prolactin to occur.

The surgical procedure and experimental protocol were the same as described by Bond, Pasley, Koike, and Llerena (this volume) with the exception that a group of 15 sexually mature male rats underwent bilateral adrenalectomy 10 days prior to the experiment. Following adrenalectomy, the animals were maintained on a 1% NaCl, 1% glucose drinking water solution in addition to the standard diet of Purina Rat Chow. Three days prior to the experiment the rats received an intramuscular injection of dexamethasone (Decadron Phosphate, Merck Sharp and Dohme) once daily at a dose of 50 µg/100 gm of body weight to ensure adequate urine flow (Weiderholt and Weiderholt, 1968). On the day of the experiment, the adrenalectomized rats were divided into a saline-treated group consisting of 7 rats each of which received a 0.2 ml

TABLE 1: THE EFFECT OF PROLACTIN ON URINE FLOW AND URINARY OSMO-
LALITY IN ADRENALECTOMIZED MALE RATS

	n	Urine Flow (% of control) Time in Minutes -15 / 0 / 15 / 30 / 45 / 60	Osmolality (% of control) Time in Minutes -15 / 0 / 15 / 30 / 45 / 60
Saline	7	100 100 108 120 114 99 ±1 ±1 ±12 ±19 ±17 ±10	99 101 101 100 101 114 ±2 ±2 ±9 ±12 ±11 ±12
Prolactin	8	100 100 70 96 95 96 ±7 ±7 ±4 ±5 ±4 ±9	101 99 143 116 113 117 ±1 ±1 ±10 ±8 ±7 ±6
p		.02	.006

Values represent means and their standard errors

intravenous injection of saline and a prolactin treated group consisting of 8 rats each of which received an intravenous injection of 20 µg of ovine prolactin (NIH).

The results of this experiment are seen in Tables 1 and 2. Prolactin significantly reduced urine flow in adrenalectomized rats 15 minutes postinjection (Table 1). Urine osmolality also was significantly increased at 15 minutes after injection of prolactin (Table 1). Sodium excretion was not different between groups while potassium excretion was significantly greater in the prolactin-treated rats 45 minutes after injection (Table 2). The effects of prolactin on urine flow, osmolality, and sodium excretion were essentially the same as seen in normal intact rats.

TABLE 2: THE EFFECT OF PROLACTIN ON SODIUM EXCRETION AND POTAS-
SIUM EXCRETION IN ADRENALECTOMIZED MALE RATS

	n	Sodium Excretion (% of control) Time in Minutes -15 / 0 / 15 / 30 / 45 / 60	Potassium Excretion (% of control) Time in Minutes -15 / 0 / 15 / 30 / 45 / 60
Saline	7	97 103 115 130 132 139 ±4 ±2 ±6 ±12 ±19 ±14	100 100 103 100 85 93 ±4 ±4 ±6 ±8 ±5 ±8
Prolactin	8	97 103 123 128 128 151 ±3 ±3 ±11 ±11 ±13 ±25	99 101 106 114 107 123 ±3 ±3 ±7 ±9 ±10 ±22
p			.04

Values represent means and their standard error

Since the effects on urine flow, osmolality, and sodium excretion in adrenalectomized male rats were not different from those seen in normal intact rats, the adrenal gland is apparently not required for the antidiuretic effect of prolactin.

The reason for the significant potassium loss seen in adrenalectomized rats 45 minutes after prolactin injection is not known. One explanation, however, may be that in the adrenalectomized rat, prolactin induced an increased delivery of sodium to the distal tubule exchange site which resulted in the observed kaluresis.

In conclusion, our results indicate that the adrenal apparently does not play a major role in the antidiuretic effect of prolactin on the kidney.

REFERENCES

Burstyn, P.G., Horrobin, D.F., and Manku, M.S. (1972). Saluretic action of aldosterone in the presence of increased salt intake and restoration of normal action by prolactin or by oxytocin. J. Endocrinol. 55, 369-376.

Horrobin, D.F., Manku, M.S., and Burstyn, P.G. (1973). Saluretic action of aldosterone in the presence of excess cortisol: Restoration of salt-retaining action of prolactin. J. Endocrinol. 56, 343-344.

Relkin, R., and Adachi, M. (1973). Effects of sodium deprivation on pituitary and plasma prolactin, growth hormone, and thyrotropin levels in the rat. Neuroendocrinology 11, 240-247.

Weiderholt, M., and Weiderholt, B. (1968). Influence of dexamethasone on water and electrolyte excretion in adrenalectomized rats. Pflugers Archiv 302, 57-58.

ACKNOWLEDGEMENTS

The prolactin used in this experiment was kindly supplied by the National Institute of Arthritis and Metabolic Disease.

This study was supported in part by Grant HL 16303 from the National Institutes of Health.

ADDENDUM

Since completing these studies, the ovine prolactin preparation (NIH SP10) has been assayed for ADH activity. Dr. Gary L. Robertson (Indianapolis, Indiana) performed the radioimmunoassay and found that 2012 ± 265 microunits (mean ± SD) of ADH were present per milligram of prolactin. The 20 µg of prolactin injected in the rats, therefore, would contain approximately 40 microunits of ADH. This amount of ADH is sufficient to account for the decline of urine flow in the normal rats following the injection of prolactin. Also, it would explain why there was no decrease in urine flow 15 minutes after prolactin injection in the ADH-loaded rats. In our experiments, therefore, it would appear that the renal response produced by the intravenous injection of ovine prolactin is most likely due to the presence of ADH in the ovine prolactin and not to the effects of prolactin.

THE EFFECT OF ERGOCORNINE ON WATER AND SODIUM METABOLISM IN

FEMALE RATS

T.I. Koike, G.C. Bond, J.N. Pasley, and L. Llerena

Department of Physiology and Biophysics
University of Arkansas Medical Center
Little Rock, AR   72201

Although the role of prolactin in modifying the excretion of sodium and water in mammals has not been extensively studied, the intraperitoneal (ip) administration of exogenous prolactin in the rat results in renal retention of salt and water (Lockett and Nail, 1965). These observations raise the possibility that endogenous variations in prolactin levels might conceivably influence the turnover of sodium and water in this species. We have examined this question using sexually mature female rats because of the known changes in serum prolactin levels that occur with each estrus cycle (Meites, Lu, Wuttke, Welsch, Nagasawa, and Quadri, 1972). The data to be presented here compares sodium and water balance prior to and during treatment with ergocornine, an alkaloid which blocks the rise in serum prolactin levels normally observed during proestrous and estrus in rats (Meites *et al.*, 1972).

Nine female Sprague-Dawley rats weighing 250 to 290 gm were placed in individual metabolism cages in an environmentally controlled room. The relative humidity was 54 ± 0.5% (mean ± S.E.) and room temperature was 71.6 ± 0.3°C. They were offered deionized water and a purified diet containing 215 µEq Na and 125 µEq K per gm. Vaginal smears were made to select normally cycling rats, and the rats were adapted for 10 days to the cages, purified diet, and the daily experimental protocol before observations were begun. Sodium and water balance were evaluated by daily measurement of body weight, food and water intake, and urinary and fecal excretion (Radford, 1959). Sodium in urine, feces, and the diet was determined by atomic absorption spectrophotometry.

After two complete estrous cycles were observed the studies were continued for an additional 2 cycles during which daily ip

Table 1. EFFECT OF ERGOCORNINE ON SODIUM TURNOVER DURING THE ESTROUS CYCLE IN RATS

		Sodium Intake μEq/day/100g	Sodium Output μEq/day/100g Urine	Sodium Output μEq/day/100g Feces	Sodium Output μEq/day/100g Total	Sodium Retention μEq/day/100g
Control	Nonestrous	1286 ± 37	1018 ± 38	33 ± 4	1051 ± 39	235 ± 27
Control	Estrous	1115 ± 30	800 ± 35	34 ± 4	834 ± 36	281 ± 35
	p	<.001	<.001	n.s.	<.001	<.05
Ergocornine	Nonestrous	1119 ± 36	820 ± 35	36 ± 8	856 ± 39	262 ± 29
Ergocornine	Estrous	997 ± 45	611 ± 35	35 ± 6	646 ± 34	331 ± 35
	p	<.001	<.001	n.s.	<.001	n.s.

Values represent mean ± standard error
Number of animals = 9
n.s. = not significant ($p<.05$)

Table 2. EFFECT OF ERGOCORNINE ON WATER TURNOVER DURING THE ESTROUS CYCLE IN RATS

		Water Intake ml/day/100g Drunk	Preformed	Oxidation	Total	Water Output ml/day/100g Urine	Feces	Insensible	Total	Water Retention ml/day/100g
Control	Nonestrous	8.12 ±0.76	0.46 ±0.01	2.29 ±0.07	10.85 ±0.81	5.18 ±0.65	0.25 ±0.02	3.69 ±0.12	9.20 ±0.72	1.66 ±0.20
Control	Estrous	7.74 ±0.69	0.39 ±0.01	1.98 ±0.05	10.12 ±0.73	4.31 ±0.61	0.25 ±0.01	3.25 ±0.09	7.83 ±0.66	2.28 ±0.23
	p	n.s.	<.005	<.001	<.002	<.005	n.s.	<.001	<.005	<.001
Ergocornine	Nonestrous	8.78 ±1.06	0.39 ±0.01	1.98 ±0.07	10.83 ±1.07	5.78 ±0.93	0.23 ±0.03	3.28 ±0.11	9.26 ±0.90	1.53 ±0.24
Ergocornine	Estrous	7.92 ±1.08	0.34 ±0.02	1.74 ±0.08	9.96 ±1.10	5.02 ±0.97	0.22 ±0.02	2.87 ±0.13	8.10 ±1.01	1.90 ±0.22
	p	n.s.	<.005	<.005	n.s.	<<.05	n.s.	<.005	<.01	n.s.

Values represent mean ± standard error
Number of animals = 9
n.s. = not significant ($p<.05$)

injections of 0.2 mg ergocornine were given. The metabolic data were divided into two categories: estrous and nonestrous. "Estrous" refers to data collected during proestrous and estrous while "nonestrous" refers to metestrous and diestrous stages of the cycle. Student's t-test for paired observations was used to evaluate the data.

The effect of ergocornine on sodium balance is summarized in Table 1. Sodium intake and excretion (urine and feces) were significantly greater during nonestrous than in estrous both during the control period and during ergocornine treatment. Retention of sodium during the control period was significantly higher during estrous than during nonestrous whereas no statistically significant differences were noted between the two stages with ergocornine treatment.

The water balance data are shown in Table 2. Total water intake was significantly different between nonestrous and estrous stages during the control period but not during ergocornine treatment. Significant differences in water output between nonestrous and estrous stages were noted both during control and ergocornine treatment. Water retention was significantly higher during the estrous stage in control but no statistically significant differences were found during ergocornine treatment.

These results show that ergocornine attenuates the increase in retention of sodium and water during estrus in the rat. The appearance of vaginal cornification and the cyclic depression in food intake indicate that the rise in estrogen levels during estrus was not blocked by the alkaloid. The suppression of water and sodium retention during estrus in ergocornine-treated rats would suggest that prolactin may play a role in causing the increase in retention of sodium and water during estrus in this species.

REFERENCES

Lockett, M.F. and Nail, B. (1965). A comparative study of the renal actions of growth and lactogenic hormones in rats. J. Physiol. 180, 146-156.

Meites, J., Lu, K.H., Wuttke, W., Welsch, C.W., Nagasawa, H., and Quadri, S.K. (1972). Recent studies on functions and control of prolactin in rats. Recent Prog. Horm. Res. 28, 471-526.

Radford, E.P. Jr. (1959). Factors modifying water metabolism in rats fed dry diets. Am. J. Physiol. 196, 1098-1108.

Acknowledgement: Ergocornine (Batch #00701) was generously provided by Sandoz Pharmaceuticals.

This study was supported in part by Grant HL 16303 from the National Institutes of Health.

DISCUSSION AFTER SHORT PRESENTATIONS

Dr. Mills

Have you excluded the possibility that your prolactin preparations contain some ADH?

Dr. Bond

No, we have not. The ovine prolactin preparation was obtained through the NIH hormone distribution program. It was not stated in the information which was forwarded with the prolactin if the preparation was assayed for either antidiuretic activity or pressor activity. Therefore, we cannot exclude the possibility that some ADH was present in the ovine prolactin.

Dr. Mills

That prolactin is made in our laboratories, and I don't know either what they do about ADH; I don't think it is assayed for that. We have found it contaminating some preparations of human growth hormone in quantities that were troublesome in some systems. Usually it is not a problem. Strangely enough, with monkey growth hormone contamination with ADH is a real problem. When you assay some preparations of monkey growth hormone by the weight gain test, the rats' paws and ears often become very white from the vasopressor effect. There must be some oxytocin there too. We've had pigeons die soon after an injection, which I suppose was due to a lowering of blood pressure. Ion exchange chromatography should remove any of that type of contamination; but most of the prolactin that's distributed has not been through ion exchange chromatography.

Dr. Bond

So there is a possibility, then, that we may be dealing with a contaminant?

Dr. Mills

I think it's a possibility worth excluding.

Dr. Jacobs

I should like to amplify on Dr. Mills' comments. Dr. Leichter, working in Dr. Chase's lab in St. Louis, has found that preparations of bovine growth hormone, supplied via the NIH distribution program, were quite potent in activating bovine renal medullary adenyl cyclase. After numerous control experiments, including careful dialysis studies, he was able to determine that this activity could be entirely accounted for by the really very small degree of contamination by vasopressin which was detected by radioimmunoassay. (The vasopressin radioimmunoassays were carried out by Dr. Gary Robertson.) This is a very substantial problem because vasopressin is so potent on a weight basis, and it gains in relevance when one is

DISCUSSION

dealing with pharmacologic doses of prolactin, as in the experiments reported by Dr. Bond. One has to be extraordinarily circumspect in the interpretation of results like these, since contamination by vasopressin in the range of one part in one million by weight can account for all the adenyl cyclase stimulating activity found in microgram quantities of growth hormone.

Dr. Bond
   Yes, I agree. Do you recall the concentration of ADH found by Robertson in the growth hormone preparation?

Dr. Jacobs
   No, I do not remember the precise figure. Dr. Leichter's work was presented at the Endocrine Society meetings in June 1974 and will be published in Biochim, Biophys. Acta. Dr. Robertson, Dr. Leichter, or Dr. Chase could give you that information, which is obviously important for you to know.

Dr. Bond
   The experimental preparation used in these experiments was designed originally for use in the bioassay of ADH (Goetz, Bond, Hermreck, and Trank, 1970). Generally as little as 2.5 to 5 microunits of ADH could be detected. I agree, therefore, that a slight contamination of the ovine prolactin with ADH could influence our results and that it is important for us to rule out the possibility of contamination.

Dr. Parsons
   We've had experiences similar to those reported by others in that some of the materials we have received from the NIH contained interesting impurities. In this particular case monkey anti-rat growth hormone antiserum also appeared to contain antibodies directed against neurophysins. By use of this antiserum in our immunocytochemical studies on rat GH we have been able to reveal the neurons of the supraoptic and paraventricular nuclei in the hypothalamus. Thus, the possibility exists, I am sure, that some of the NIAMDD materials contain contaminants.

Dr. Bond
   It would appear from this discussion that an examination of the ovine prolactin preparation from NIH for contamination with ADH must be thoroughly conducted before any final conclusions can be made concerning the role of exogenously administered prolactin in influencing the renal excretion of salt and water.

QUESTION: Has anybody looked at the effect of prolactin on renin activity?

Dr. Pasley
   I am not aware of any direct evidence concerning prolactin

and renin levels. On the other hand, I would invite your attention to work by Lawson and Gala (1974), who found significant increases in plasma prolactin levels after blood volume reduction in ovariectomized rats and by Relkin, Adachi, and Kahan (1972), who noted increased pituitary and plasma prolactin levels in rats maintained on a sodium deficient diet. Both studies are suggestive of enhanced renin production in association with increased prolactin production. Specific data, however, are not yet available, although we hope to explore this point.

Dr. Fleming

This is, in a way, sort of strange to me because I've worked with fish primarily throughout most of my life and prolactin is so terribly potent and so important in regulating sodium and water metabolism in a wide variety of teleosts. I've been very interested in what you have to say because it was sort of disappointing to me that it doesn't have nearly as important a role in the higher vertebrates. I'd also say, and once again this is based on my own selfish interests, I'm surprised that this hasn't been looked at a lot more.

Dr. Koike

The action of prolactin on the mammalian kidney has been studied by Lockett (1965; Lockett and Nail, 1965) and by Horrobin's group in England (Burstyn, Horrobin, and Manku, 1972; Horrobin, Manku, and Burstyn, 1973). In a recent review (Nicoll and Bern, 1972), it was suggested that prolactin would appear to have a sodium retaining action on the mammalian kidney. We became interested in the renal action of prolactin following the report that the mammalian kidney possesses receptors specific for prolactin (Turkington, 1972), *viz.*, whether this hormone might influence the excretion of sodium and/or water. Renal physiologists have, particularly over the past 10 to 15 years, been searching for a third, or other factors besides renal hemodynamics and aldosterone to explain the regulation of sodium balance. This is the reason we decided to look at extrinsic humoral factors which might influence sodium excretion by the mammalian kidney.

Dr. Fleming

Thank you. I know that Professor J.O. Davis on this campus has been doing that, and I won't tell him about your results on this.

DISCUSSION REFERENCES

Burstyn, P.G., Horrobin, D.F., and Manku, M.S. (1972). Saluretic action of aldosterone in the presence of increased salt intake and restoration of normal action by prolactin or by oxytocin. J. Endocrinol. 55, 369-376.

DISCUSSION

Goetz, K.L., Bond, G.C., Hermreck, A.S., and Trank, J.W. (1970). Plasma ADH levels following a decrease in mean atrial transmural pressure in dogs. Am. J. Physiol. 219, 1424-1428.

Horrobin, D.F., Manku, M.S., and Burstyn, P.G. (1973). Saluretic action of aldosterone in the presence of excess cortisol: Restoration of salt-retaining action by prolactin. J. Endocrinol. 56, 343-344.

Lawson, D.M. and Gala, R.R. (1974). The influence of surgery, time of day, blood volume reduction and anaesthetics on plasma prolactin in ovariectomized rats. J. Endocrinol. 62, 75-83.

Lockett, M.F. (1965). Comparison of the direct renal actions of pituitary growth and lactogenic hormones. J. Physiol. 181, 192-199.

Lockett, M.F. and Nail, B. (1965). A comparative study of the renal actions of growth and lactogenic hormones in rats. J. Physiol. 180, 146-156.

Nicoll, C.S. and Bern, H.A. (1972). On the actions of prolactin amont the vertebrates: Is there a common denominator? In: *Lactogenic Hormones* (Wolstenholme, G.E.W. and Knight, J., eds.), pp 299-324, Churchill Livingstone, Edinburgh and London.

Relkin, R., Adachi, M., and Kahan, S.A. (1972). Effects of pinealectomy and constant light and darkness on prolactin levels in the pituitary and plasma and on pituitary ultrastructure of the rat. J. Endocrinol. 54, 263-268.

Turkington, R.W. (1972). Human prolactin, an ancient molecule provides new insight for clinical medicine. Am. J. Med. 53, 389-394.

SUBJECT INDEX

Acetylcholine, prolactin release, 146
Adrenal cortical hormones, lactation, 5, 7, 10, 146, 174, 179
    mammary growth, 180
    milk production, 181
    natriuresis, prolactin-induced, 197-200
    pituitary prolactin, 7, 8
Adrenergic pathways and prolactin release, 9
Age,
    fat stores, 155
    pituitary prolactin, 5
Aldosterone,
    mammary growth, 179
    milk production, 10
Alveolar proliferation, 179
Amniotic fluid prolactin, 26
Amphibian metamorphosis, 152
Androgens and mammary growth, 180, 181
Anesthetics and prolactin release, 9, 10, 132
Annual cycles in fat stores, 155-158
Assay of prolactin, 2, 6, 8, 11
Atropine and prolactin release, 9

Big prolactin, 103, 104, 106
Bovine,
    growth hormone and lactation, 130
    mammotrophs, 38
    milk production, 9, 11
    pituitary prolactin, 5
    prolactin and lactation, 129, 130
    prolactin storage granules, 50
    prolactin structure, 23-25
Breast cancer,
    prolactin, 131
    reserpine, 130
Breast stimulation and prolactin release, 106-109, 181

Calciferol and milk production, 10
Catecholamines,
    lactation, 138
    prolactin release, 53, 54, 87, 138, 139, 151, 177, 178
Cattle (see Bovine)
Chiari-Frommel syndrome, 146
Cholinergic drugs and prolactin release, 139, 142
Cholinergic pathways and prolactin release, 9
Chorionic somatomammotropin,
    mammogenesis, 174, 181
    milk production, 181
    oxidation, 29
Circadian rhythms and the fattening response to prolactin, 158-161
Corticosterone and mild production, 10
Crinophagy of prolactin granules, 44, 52, 53, 66, 67, 86, 88, 90-92
Crop sac (see Pigeon crop sac)

Dibenamine and prolactin release, 9
Diethylstilbestrol,
    lactation, 6, 7, 9
    pituitary prolactin, 6, 8
    prolactin release, 177

Dissociated cells and prolactin release, 41
Dog, prolactin and lactation, 2
L-Dopa,
    lactation, 146, 147, 151
    prolactin release, 131, 138, 139, 143, 145, 176
Dopamine and prolactin release, 114-119, 176, 178

Endoplasmic reticulum in mammotrophs, 39, 44-47, 58-61, 70, 71, 93
Electrolyte metabolism and prolactin, 170
Entrainment of circadian rhythms of fattening responses to prolactin,
    adrenal corticosteroids, 162-164, 166
    daily photoperiod, 161, 162
    hypophysectomy, 165
    thyroxine, 165, 166
Ergot alkaloids,
    prolactin-induced natriuresis, 201-203
    prolactin release, 145, 146
    prolactin release inhibitory factor (PIF), 145
Estradiol and placentoma formation, 11
Estrogens,
    lactation, 6, 11, 181, 182
    mammary growth, 174, 177, 179-181
    milk production, 178
    pituitary prolactin, 2, 5-8, 135
    prolactin release, 53, 55, 144-146, 177
Estrus and pituitary prolactin, 135
Exercise and plasma prolactin, 110, 111
Exocytosis of prolactin granules, 50-52, 65, 88, 89

Fat stores,
    age variations, 155
    annual cycles, 155-158
    daily photoperiod, 156, 157
    handling disturbances, 166, 167, 170, 171
    migration, 155-158
    prolactin influences, 158
    seasonal changes, 155-158
Fattening responses to prolactin,
    circadian variations, 158-161
    entrainment, 161-166
Follicle stimulating hormone release from prolactin, 151
Food consumption and prolactin, 160
Forbes-Albright syndrome, 146
Free water clearance and prolactin, 195

Galactin (also see prolactin), 1-3
Galactorrhea, 120, 121, 128, 183 185, 187
Goat, prolactin and lactation, 7, 8
Golden top-minnow, 154, 155, 160, 161, 165, 166
Golgi apparatus in mammotrophs, 38, 39, 44-48, 57-59, 62-64, 68, 69, 74, 75, 93
Green anole lizard, 155, 156, 162, 164, 167
Growth hormone,
    lactation in cattle, 130
    mammary growth, 179, 180
    milk production, 9, 10
    oxidation, 29
    pigeon crop sac activity, 130
    prolactin activity, 32-34, 97-100
    suckling, 139
Guinea pig,
    lactation, 2, 5
    pituitary prolactin, 3, 7
Gulf killifish, 162, 164

Hagfish, 24, 34

INDEX

Handling,
    fat stores, 166, 167, 170, 171
    plasma chloride, 170
History of prolactin, 1-17
Hog prolactin and lactation, 2
Human prolactin, chemistry, 24, 25
Hypoglycemia and prolactin, 110
Hypophysectomy,
    entrainment of circadian responses to prolactin, 165
    lactation, 5
Hypothalamus and prolactin release, 53, 135-138, 142-144, 147, 174-177

Insulin,
    lactogenesis, 174, 179
    milk production, 10, 181
    prolactin release, 146

Japanese quail, 167

Kangaroo, 191

Lactation,
    adrenocortical hormones, 5, 7, 10, 146, 174, 179
    catecholamines, 138
    diethylstilbestrol, 6, 7
    L-Dopa, 146, 147, 151
    estrogens, 6, 11, 181, 182
    hypophysectomy, 5
    insulin, 174, 179
    monoamine oxidase inhibitors, 138
    pregnancy, 4, 5, 7
    progesterone, 182
    prolactin, 2, 5, 173-192
    testosterone, 6
    thyroid, 5, 174
    thyrotropin, 5
Lactogenesis,
    adrenocortical hormones, 174, 179
    estrogens, 181, 182
    insulin, 174, 179
    progesterone, 182
    prolactin, 173-192
    thyroid, 174
Lamprey, 24, 34
Lipid index, 154
Lipogenesis in the pigeon, 160
Liporegulation and prolactin, 153-168
Litter size and pituitary prolactin, 4
Luteotropic hormone release and prolactin, 151
Luetotropin releasing hormone and prolactin, 146

Male, prolactin, 2, 131, 132
Mammary tumors, 146, 147
Mammogenesis,
    adrenal steroids, 179, 180
    alveolar proliferation, 179
    androgens, 180, 181
    chorionic somatomammotropin, 181
    estrogens, 174, 177, 179, 180, 181
    growth hormone, 179, 180
    placental hormones, 174
    pregnancy, 181
    progesterone, 174, 179-181
    prolactin, 173-192
    thyroid, 180
Mammotrophs,
    bovine, 38
    crinophagy, 44
    Golgi apparatus, 38, 39, 44-48, 57-59, 62-64, 68, 69, 74, 75, 93
    identification, 37-39, 57, 68, 69
    polyribosomes, 41, 44-46, 58, 59
    rat, 38, 57
    rough endoplasmic reticulum, 39, 44-47, 58-61, 70, 71, 93
    secretory granules, 38, 44, 45, 47, 48, 57, 62-65, 76, 77
Menstrual cycle prolactin variations, 190
Migration and fat stores, 155-158

Milk, prolactin content, 183, 184
Milk composition, 5
Milk production,
adrenal hormones, 10, 181
aldosterone, 10
calciferol, 10
chorionic somatomammo-
tropin, 181
corticosterone, 10
diethylstilbestrol, 9
estrogens, 178
growth hormone, 9, 10
insulin, 10, 181
oral contraceptives, 178
parathyroid hormones, 10
prolactin, 10, 11, 181
thyroid hormones, 9, 10, 181
Monkey, lactation, 2
Monoamine oxidase inhibitors and lactation, 138
Mouse, 2, 3, 7, 167
Mouse breast culture, prolactin assay, 95-99

Natriuresis, 193-203
Nembutal and prolactin release, 1, 10, 146
Nursing (see suckling)

Oral contraceptives,
milk production, 178
prolactin release, 177, 178
Osmolality of plasma and prolactin release, 112, 166
Ovariectomy and pituitary prolactin, 6
Ovine prolactin, chemistry, 23-25
Oxytocin and prolactin release, 9, 10, 146

Parathyroid hormones and milk production, 10
Parturition, pituitary prolactin, 135
Pentobarbital and prolactin release, 9, 10, 146

Photoperiod,
entrainment of circadian responses to prolactin, 161, 162
fat stores, 156, 157
Pigeon, 162, 165
lipogenesis, 160
pituitary prolactin, 8
Pigeon crop sac,
prolactin assay, 2, 6, 8, 11, 95
growth hormone activity, 130
Pituitary tumors, 120-122, 128
Placental lactogen (see chorionic somatomammotropin)
Placentoma formation, 11
Postpartum pituitary prolactin, 2, 3
Potassium excretion, urinary, 193-200
Polyribosomes in mammotrophs, 41, 44-46, 58, 59
Porcine prolactin, chemistry, 23-25
Pregnancy,
lactation, 4, 5, 7
mammary growth, 181
pituitary prolactin, 2-4, 7, 135
prolactin release, 112, 177
urinary prolactin, 6
Progesterone,
lactogenesis, 182
mammogenesis, 174, 179-181
pituitary prolactin, 7, 8
prolactin release, 146
Propranolol and prolactin release, 150, 151
Prolactin,
assay, 2, 6, 8, 11, 95-102
cellular actions, 8
electrolyte metabolism, 170
fat stores, 158
food consumption, 160
follicle stimulating hormone release, 151
free water clearance, 195
granules, exocytosis, and crinophagy, 50-53, 65-67, 86, 88-92

INDEX

historical perspectives, 1-17
lactation, 2, 129, 130
lactogenesis, 173-192
luteinizing hormone release, 151
male, 131, 132
mammogenesis, 173-192
milk composition, 5
milk concentration, 183, 184
milk production, 181
milk secretion, 10, 11
natriuresis, 197-203
placentoma formation, 11
storage granules, 49, 50, 57
cellular events, 41-50
urinary, 6, 30, 31
urine osmolality, 193-199
urinary sodium and potassium excretion, 193-203
water balance, 201-203
Prolactin, chemistry, 19-35
aggregation, 22
amnionic fluid, 26
"big" and "little" prolactin, 103, 104, 106
chemical modifications, 23
deamidation, 21, 22, 31
enzymatic alteration, 22, 23
extraction, 19, 20, 30
oxidation, 29
physicochemical properties, 23
polymerization, 22, 31, 32
primary structure, 23-25
purification, 19-21
Prolactin, pituitary content,
adrenocortical hormones, 7, 8
age differences, 5
diethylstilbestrol, 6, 8
estrogens, 2, 5-8, 135
estrus, 135
litter size, 4
ovariectomy, 6
parturition, 135
postpartum, 2, 3
pregnancy, 2-4, 7, 135
progesterone, 6-8
sex differences, 3, 5, 8
suckling, 3, 9
testosterone, 6, 8
thiouracil, 8, 135
thyroidectomy, 8, 135
Prolactin, release and secretion,
acetylcholine, 146
adrenergic pathways, 9
anesthetics, 9, 10, 132, 146
atropine, 9
breast stimulation, 106, 107, 109, 181
catecholamines, 53, 54, 87, 138, 139, 151, 177, 178
cellular mechanisms, 40-55
cholinergic drugs, 139, 142
cholinergic pathways, 9
dibenamine, 9
diethylstilbestrol, 177
dissociated cells, 41
L-Dopa, 138, 139, 143, 145, 176
dopamine, 114-119
ergot drugs, 145, 146
estrogens, 53, 55, 112, 113, 144-146, 177
exercise, 110, 111
hypoglycemia, 110
hypothalamic factors, 53, 135-138, 142-144, 147, 174-176
insulin, 146
luteotropin releasing hormone, 146
menstrual cycle, 190
monamine oxidase inhibitors, 138
oral contraceptives, 177, 179
oxytocin, 9, 10, 146
pentobarbital, 9, 10, 146
plasma osmolality, 112, 166
pregnancy, 112, 177
progesterone, 146
prolactin releasing factor, 54, 86
prolactin release inhibiting

factor, 54, 86, 136-138, 179
propranolol, 150, 151
prostaglandins, 138, 142
psychic factors, 127, 128
puerperium, 182
reserpine, 178
serotonin, 138, 142, 143, 177
sexual intercourse, 111, 112
sleep, 108-111
somatostatin, 139, 141, 146
stress, 109, 110, 144
suckling, 106, 107, 139, 140, 144
temperature, 146
thyroid, 113, 178
thyrotropin releasing hormone, 54, 87, 113-115, 138, 142-145, 175-177
thyroxine, 53, 145
vasopressin, 146
Prolactin, plasma levels (also see prolactin, release, and secretion),
humans, 104-114
menstrual cycle variations, 190
pituitary tumors, 120-122, 128
pregnancy, 112, 177
puerperium, 182
sex differences, 104, 105, 129
sleep, 108-111
temperature, 142, 143
Prolactin releasing factor, 54, 86
Prolactin release inhibiting factor, 54, 86, 136-138, 145, 179
Prostaglandins, 138, 142
Prostate and prolactin, 131, 132
Paychic factors and prolactin release, 127, 128

Puerperium, 182

Rabbit, 1-5, 7, 8
Radioimmunoassay of prolactin, 99-102
Rat, 2, 3, 6, 8-11, 38, 50, 57, 193-206
Reserpine,
breast cancer, 130
oxytocin release, 10
prolactin release, 178
Rough endoplasmic reticulum, 39, 44-47, 58-61, 70, 71, 93

Secretory granules in mammotrophs, 38, 44, 45, 47, 48, 56, 62-65, 76, 77
Serotonin, 138, 142, 143, 177
Sex differences in pituitary prolactin, 3, 5, 8
Sexual intercourse and prolactin release, 111, 112
Shark prolactin, chemistry, 23, 24
Sheep, 1, 23, 25
Sleep, prolactin levels, 108-111
Sodium excretion, 193-203
Somatostatin and prolactin release, 139, 141, 146
Sow (see hog)
Storage granules of prolactin, 49, 50, 57
Stress, prolactin release, 109, 110, 144
Sturgeon growth hormone, 34, 35
Suckling,
growth hormone release, 139
pituitary prolactin, 3, 9
prolactin release, 106, 107, 139, 140, 144

Temperature and prolactin release, 142, 143
Testosterone,
lactation, 6
pituitary prolactin, 6, 8
prolactin release, 146
Thiouracil and pituitary prolactin, 8, 135
Thyroid hormones,
lactogenesis, 174

mammary growth, 180
milk production, 181
prolactin release, 113, 178
Thyroidectomy and pituitary prolactin, 8, 135
Thyrotropin and lactation, 5
Thyrotropin releasing hormone and prolactin release, 54, 87, 113-115, 138, 142-145, 175-177
Thyroxine,
    entrainment of circadian responses to prolactin, 165, 166
    lactation, 5
    milk production, 9, 10
    prolactin release, 53, 145

Urine osmolality, 193-199

Vasopressin and prolactin release, 146

Water balance and prolactin, 201-203
Whale prolactin, chemistry, 24, 25
White-crowned sparrow, 158-160
White-throated sparrow, 155-160, 162, 164